3 Steps to Gluten-Free Living

3 Steps to Gluten-Free Living

—\\\—

*A Practical Step-By-Step Guide to the **Elimination, Transition**, and **Substitution** of Gluten to Promote Healing and Health for Life*

Gluten-Free Bebe™

Melinda Arcara

ISBN: 1512188751
ISBN 13: 9781512188752
Library of Congress Control Number: 2015907796
CreateSpace Independent Publishing Platform
North Charleston, South Carolina

Table of Contents

Introduction

Whether you have decided to go gluten-free or you have been diagnosed with celiac disease or a gluten intolerance, you are now faced with this question:

"Where do I start?"

Going gluten-free is as easy as one, two, three; you just have to take it step by step. This book is your practical guide to help you understand what gluten is, where it is found, and how to change your eating habits by following three simple steps:

- **Elimination** of gluten 100 percent from your diet.
- **Transition** your home and family to a new way of eating.
- **Substitution** of delicious gluten-free foods, products, ingredients, and recipes to help you stay compliant and feel better quickly.

3 Steps to Gluten-Free Living

The faster you learn these three steps, the more compliant you will become, the quicker your body will respond, and the better you will feel.

Five years ago, after suffering from a lifetime of unexplained symptoms (diarrhea, weight fluctuations, anxiety, paranoia, brain fog, joint pain, migraines, infertility, stomach pains, gas, bloating, etc.), I was finally diagnosed with a gluten intolerance. In my world, this news was a blessing, not a curse.

When I think back over my life, I'm amazed at how sick I was for such a long time. As a matter of fact, my journey probably started when I was very young. I am the youngest of ten children, or as my dad would say, the "bebe" (pronounced bee-bee) of the family. I grew up on wonderful Eastern European foods like pierogis, nut rolls, and every baked good my Slovak mum could make. With ten children to feed, she was rarely out of the kitchen.

It's easy to look back now and see all the problems I had growing up with learning, attention, and behavior. I couldn't keep my eyes on the pages of assigned books, so reading long books was almost impossible. I did poorly on standardized tests and couldn't retain information I had just learned. Back in the 1980s, no one took the time to figure out why I was a mediocre student, probably because I had a very BIG personality to distract people from my grades. My humor was my crutch. I knew I wasn't stupid; I could learn from someone speaking information, but I couldn't open a book and comprehend concepts on my own. I shudder knowing that I went through high school and four years of college without reading a novel from end to end. I was never at the top of my class academically, but with hard work, I did graduate college in four years. I am a living example that when you have love and family support (primary nutrition), your dietary nutrition (secondary nutrition) can be out of balance, and you can survive (Rosenthal 2007).

It was when I was about fourteen years old that I began to pass blood in my stool. I was given a sigmoidoscopy and diagnosed with an autoimmune problem. It was given the general name of irritable bowel syndrome (IBS), but I had no answer to what was causing the irritation. After that first sigmoidoscopy, the doctors explained to me that the IBS would slowly move through my intestines and "eventually turn to colitis and perhaps colon cancer." It was a scary thing to explain to a fourteen-year-old. I spent the next six years hiding symptoms from my mum or refusing to see doctors for fear of the embarrassment of the procedure preps and the mention of a colonoscopy, which at the time required a longer hospital stay than the sigmoidoscopy.

Every major life event from the time I turned twenty until I had my daughter at thirty-six (college, jobs, marriage, infertility, pregnancy, death of my dad) resulted in a weakened immune system, and subsequently I would have a colonoscopy to determine if the IBS had gotten worse or turned into colitis. I was on one antibiotic after another. I went to one type of doctor and then another for different aches and pains (joint pain, bladder infections, sore throats, acne, etc.). I felt like I was always complaining about how I was feeling.

After struggling to get pregnant for four years, I finally had our son when I was thirty-four. That's when I started to get migraines with flashing auras. After having my daughter at thirty-six, they got worse, and I eventually contacted a neurologist to rule out any brain defects. All tests (CAT scans, MRIs, etc.) came back normal. He suggested that I try taking riboflavin (B2). He didn't know why it worked for some people, but I didn't want to go on prescription medicine, so this was my last resort. Thankfully, it cut the number of migraines to one or two a month. But I continued to battle with arthritic pain, foggy brain, fatigue, anxiety, and depression.

Right before my fortieth birthday, everything fell apart for me emotionally and physically. My ob-gyn suggested that I go on birth control pills to help with my remaining migraines. My physician, on the other hand, suggested I go on an antidepressant to help "even out my moods." Finally, Sue, one of my sisters, who was already gluten- and dairy-free, stepped in and found a local holistic health practitioner for me who was able to diagnose me with non-celiac gluten intolerance and a severe iron and vitamin B deficiency. Holistic health was foreign to me, so before I went on any vitamin supplements, I decided to consult my family doctor as a backup. Western medicine blood tests matched the holistic/Eastern medicine tests, so from that point I was on my way to being gluten-free.

I cried tears of joy when I finally had a diagnosis for the way I felt. It took me seven days to detox from gluten, but once I got over the cravings, I immediately noticed that I could breathe out of the right side of my nose. I bet I hadn't done that my entire life. My skin cleared, my hair and nails got thicker and stronger, and I could actually read entire books! My digestive system could finally absorb the vitamins and nutrients from the foods and supplements I was taking. It was amazing how quickly my body was healed just by eliminating gluten.

The first six months were a learning process. I wasn't quite sure what products contained gluten, so I would inadvertently go on and off gluten, feeling sick each time I ingested something I shouldn't. Reading labels and trying to decipher gluten-containing ingredients in foods in my pantry was a huge stress. I found that I would eat junk food, like potato chips, because I didn't know what else I could safely eat, or I wouldn't eat at all. By the seventh month, I made the full commitment to stay gluten-free, and I began to realize it was not only about the *elimination* of foods from my pantry but also about the *substitution* of naturally gluten-free foods.

With that new realization, I began to fill my pantry with anything and everything I could find with a gluten-free label and spent way too much money in the process. It was a slow and emotional process, and I vowed that I would help other people become gluten-free more easily (and cheaply) than I did. Since then, I have helped many people with my three-step approach to becoming gluten-free, so they can feel better quickly and save time and money in the process. Also, and a very important point I want to state up front, eating gluten-free, if not done correctly, can be much less healthy for you. Substituting the right ingredients and eating clean and whole are what I stress and teach you in this book.

This book is a hands-on, practical guide to help you organize your home and heart with simple, thought-provoking exercises, tips, facts, and recipes with spaces on each page to keep notes each time you find new information you want to remember. Each page is a new topic and another step toward becoming 100 percent gluten-free. You'll want to keep this book as your personal reference guide, so be sure to write in pencil as products, prices, thoughts, and information change quickly in the gluten-free world.

By purchasing this book, you are no longer left with the question, where do I start? Instead, go ahead and turn the pages of *3 Steps to Gluten-Free Living*, and be sure to keep your own notes on the pages provided as a reference of what works and doesn't work in your gluten-free journey. By the end of the book, you'll be ready to be 100 percent gluten-free and on your way to feeling better.

Step 1

Elimination

What is Gluten?

It's probably the first and most important question you should ask yourself after choosing or being advised by your doctor to become gluten-free. Knowing and learning what gluten is, where it comes from, and what it's used for helps you to understand what kind of foods it's in. You might not have thought that foods such as salad dressings and processed meats could contain gluten before you knew what gluten was and how it is used in everyday foods.

I certainly do not know everything there is about gluten, but I have done extensive research. I try to read everything I can about the subject (but not enough to drive myself crazy!). The following is enough information to get you started on your journey.

Gluten is found in the endosperm of certain grains—for example, wheat, barley, and rye. It is made up of two proteins, gliadin and glutenin.

- Gliadin is very sticky when it becomes wet, and it is the adhesive of the two proteins (bakeinfo).
- Glutenin is the longer complex protein and is the stretchy/elastic part of the two proteins (bakeinfo).

It's not until the two proteins are combined (with the help of added water) that gluten gets its physical properties of sticky and stretchy. These two properties are what make gluten an important part of baking bread. When the two proteins are combined, gluten becomes tough, rubbery, and elastic. This gives it the ability to rise when yeast or baking powder is added to it. That's what makes it great for baking fluffy breads (bakeinfo) (Hill).

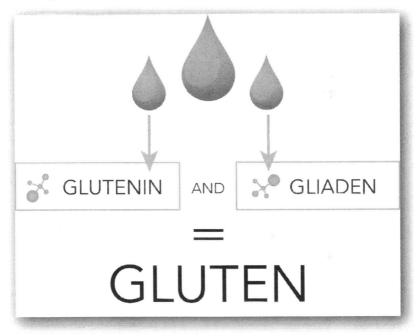

Gluten has four characteristics that are positive for baking: it absorbs two times its weight in water, it stretches, it's elastic, and it's sticky (bakeinfo). While beneficial for baking, unfortunately gluten can initiate damaging reactions in the body. When I now hear doctors talk about leaky gut, I visualize my small intestines coated with mucus and inflamed while trying to break down gluten (Hill). Leaky gut is a term used to describe the condition celiac patients suffer from when consuming gluten. The villi are fingerlike projections inside the intestinal tract that serve to absorb nutrients from food as it is passed through. When the villi are damaged from gluten exposure, the villi atrophy, or shrivel up, thus preventing nutrients from being absorbed causing nutritional deficiencies. Incompletely digested foods literally pass through the intestinal wall, along with waste and toxins, into the bloodstream. These foreign toxins trigger the body to fight itself, also called an autoimmune response.

Who Needs to Eliminate Gluten?

I'm being asked more and more by restaurant servers if I have an allergy or just intolerance. That's a sign of a savvy server or restaurant (or that the restaurant has a lot of customers asking about gluten-free options). Having an understanding of the continuum of gluten sensitivity and severity tells a restaurant a lot about what is required for safe food preparation. That shows they have a true concern for their customers' well-being.

Dr. Alessio Fazano, medical director at the University of Maryland School of Medicine's Center for Celiac Research, was the first to designate three categories of gluten intolerance (Alessio Fasano, 2013):

- Wheat or gluten allergy
- Autoimmune response (celiac or celiac sprue)
- Immune-mediated response (nonceliac gluten sensitivity)

When you think of an allergy, you think of the body's physiological response to a stimulus (e.g., gluten), and in the most severe case, an anaphylaxis reaction, which can include trouble breathing and possible need for emergency care if the reaction is severe enough. Everyone knows someone allergic to peanuts, tree nuts, shellfish, or even bees. They are always asking a lot of questions about food ingredients and perhaps even carry an EpiPen, just in case. Similar to these other allergies, a wheat or gluten allergy can have varying degrees of severity and physical reaction times (usually relatively quickly).

The second category is the autoimmune response, or celiac disease. It is diagnosed in 1 percent of the population, but there are estimates that it could be up to 10 percent because so many people could have it and not know. This autoimmune disease is diagnosed by blood tests and upper endoscopy. The lining of the small intestines is damaged, not allowing nutrients from food to be absorbed into the body. The symptoms of gluten ingestion by these people are usually slower than those of allergy sufferers. Lack of nutrition can cause symptoms of malnutrition, anemia, and slow growth in children (O'Brien 2013). It's usually associated with gastrointestinal problems (loose stools, pain, gas, etc.), but not always. Although people with celiac can feel sick immediately after ingesting gluten, many don't feel anything until malnutrition problems set in. It can take up to four years to get diagnosed with celiac because it is so silent. This is what happened to my brother-in-law when he suffered from anemia for a long time before finally being diagnosed with celiac.

Nonceliac gluten sensitivity (NCGS) is the most recent gluten-related category. Symptoms from gluten ingestion can show up days after ingestion. They are finding a wide range of symptoms all over the body (not just the digestive tract) ranging from headache, brain fog, depression, anxiety, and joint pain, to name a few (DrPerlmutter. com) (O'Brien, 2013). Currently, there are no tests to diagnose a person for NCGS. The only option is to eliminate gluten from the diet and slowly introduce it back in to see how the body responds.

If you haven't already done it, it's very important to get a proper diagnosis from your doctor or health care professional before eliminating gluten. For example, if it's celiac, knowing how much intestinal damage you have is important so the physician can monitor the body's healing. Also, having an autoimmune disorder diagnosis is important, as you have a 25 percent chance of developing additional autoimmune disorders through your life (M. Cojocaru 2010).

No matter which diagnosis or category of gluten intolerance you have, 100 percent elimination of gluten from your diet is the *only* solution to allow your body to heal from the damaging effects of gluten.

Know What Grains Contain Gluten

Becoming familiar with the many names of gluten-containing grains is a must when eating out and reading labels. It's easy to see foods that contain "alternative" grains and forget which contain gluten. It's not just wheat, barley, and rye. It's a good idea to keep the following list with you as a reference to refer to the different names of these grains.

- Barley
- Bulgur
- Couscous
- Dinkel
- Durum
- Einkorn
- Farina
- Farro
- Graham flour
- Kamut
- Matzo
- Mir
- Rye
- Seitan/Fu
- Semolina
- Spelt
- Triticale

- Oat*
- Oat bran*
- Oat fiber*
- Wheat
- Wheat germ
- Wheat grass
- Wheat berry
- Wheat nuts

*Oats contain *avenin*. They have similar amino acid sequences as wheat gluten and can evoke the immune response of celiac disease for some people. **Currently there is no way to predict ahead of time which people with celiac disease will or will not be able to successfully consume oats without an immune reaction** (CeliacSupportAssociation.com).

Why Gluten All of a Sudden?

I get this question all the time, and it's a good question. Celiac disease has been around for a long time, although it's been difficult to diagnose up until recent years. In the last five years, doctors have begun to recognize its broad array of symptoms, and they are more apt to test for gluten-related disorders than in the past. Doctors no longer stop at an irritable bowel syndrome diagnosis. Now they are looking further into what is causing the bowel irritation. In my area of the country, many people who have lethargy and headaches are being tested by their physicians for Lyme disease, and if that comes back as negative, they are tested for celiac.

I have studied three different theories behind "why gluten all of a sudden." The first theory is gluten hybridization or changes to the grain itself. Through hybridization, scientists have created a grain that is more drought resistant, insect resistant, and faster growing to meet the demands of world hunger. These changes have also added new proteins to the grains. The increased amount of protein has lengthened the shelf life of instant-gratification food like prepackaged bakery items (cakes, cookies, etc.) our society now demands. Bread that used to get moldy after several days is still palatable after many weeks. Thanks to these added proteins, shelf life has even gone to years for some products as a result of these grain modifications (McGinnis).

All this could be good for consumers because it helps keep costs down; however, the changes to these proteins have made it more difficult for our bodies to digest. The grains have changed, but our DNA hasn't had time to adapt.

The second theory is the high use of pesticides in industrialized farming. These pesticides are sprayed on crops or even into the soil they grow in. We all have heard the controversy over genetically modified organisms (GMOs), where the genes of plants are modified to carry new characteristics (herbicide tolerance and insect resistance) that support that particular product's needs. The increased use of pesticides might have damaging effects on the human digestive system, thus causing people to be unable to break down gluten. Perhaps the gut's microflorae become damaged and therefore sensitive to gluten-containing foods.

A third theory is that some wheat seeds are exposed to chemicals in a process called chemical mutagenesis, which is considered a "traditional breeding method" (nongmo-project.org). In addition to the chemicals, seeds can be exposed to gamma and x-ray radiation to induce desired mutations. This process is considered standard hybridization practice. Like GMO foods, there are no long-term studies showing this wheat product's effects on human consumption, but perhaps this new wheat might have a responsibility in the rising number of gluten intolerance sufferers.

For reference, here is a list of the most common GMO foods (http://www.nongmoproject.org/find-non-gmo/search-participating-products/):

- Alfalfa
- Corn
- Cotton
- Papaya
- Rapeseed (canola)
- Soybeans
- Sugar beets
- Tobacco
- Yellow squash
- Zucchini

Hidden Sources of Gluten

Gluten is everywhere. Not only is it found in your breads, baked goods, and snacks, but it also shows up in many unexpected products. Over the years I was often surprised that I had been eating a product containing gluten without knowing. The most recent is my dry salad dressing packet. I never dreamed it contained gluten, probably because it is a dry spice pack, but it included soy sauce in the ingredient list. Surprise!

Some other products that you might be surprised contain gluten are meats, soups, cheese products, condiments, candy and chewing gum, and toothpaste, just to name a few. Here is a list of other products that could contain gluten (Gluten Free Gluten.com) (DrPerlmutter.com).

- Baked beans (canned)
- Baking powder
- Beer
- Breading and coating mixes
- Brown rice syrup (may contain malted barley), rice products with seasoning packets
- Canned meats and fish in broth
- Cheese products: sauces, spreads, and some shredded cheeses
- Colorings

- Condiments (carefully read condiment labels as gluten is often used as a stabilizer or thickening ingredient in ketchup, mustards, and oriental sauces)
- Gum, candy, and chocolate syrup
- Deli meats, breaded fish and meats, prepackaged ground beef products, and hot dogs
- Dry-roasted nuts
- Egg mixes
- Flavorings, food starches, seasonings, and malt are vague words to watch for on packaged food labels. These terms are often clues that the product might contain gluten. For example, "malt" vinegar and "malted" milk powder contain gluten.
- Frozen french fries (in the coating)
- Gravy products (dry products, bouillon cubes, and processed, canned products)
- Ice cream and ice cream treats
- Imitation fish, meats, and cheeses
- Instant flavored coffee/cocoa mixes
- Licorice candy (black and red)
- Matzo meal
- Pickled products
- Pudding and pie fillings
- Salad dressings
- Sauces, including soy sauce, which is commonly made by fermenting wheat (Check *all* processed sauce labels—from barbeque sauce to ice cream

toppings, chili pepper products, and tomato sauce products. All may contain gluten.)

- Sausage
- Self-basting poultry products, including turkey with added "solutions"
- Snack foods, including flavored potato chips and corn chips
- Soups, stocks, and broth
- Spice and herb blends (spices and herbs in their natural form do not contain gluten)

The Different Names of Gluten

How many different names can scientists call gluten? It's no wonder our DNA hasn't caught up to the fact that there is more protein in each gluten-containing grain. Gluten is in so many of the ingredients in the Standard American Diet (SAD). When you start to look at product ingredient lists, you may see wheat, barley, or rye listed, but gluten is also found in other parts of the ingredient list. "Caramel color" or "natural flavors" are ingredients that commonly contain gluten. Small amounts of gluten start to add up when it is in three to four other ingredients. Here are just a few other names of gluten (DrPerlmutter.com) (Teri Gruss):

- Amino peptide complex
- *Avena sativa*
- Brown rice syrup
- Carmel color
- Cyclodextrin
- Dextrin
- Emulsifiers
- Extenders or thickeners
- Fermented grain extract
- Flavorings and food starches
- *Hordeum distichon*
- *Hordeum vulgare*

- Hydrolyzed vegetable protein
- Hydrolyzed food starch
- Hydrolyzed plant protein
- Hydrolyzed vegetable protein (HVP)
- Maltodextrin
- Malt (barley malt, extract or vinegar)
- Milk (if malted or flavored)
- Modified food starch
- Mono and diglycerides
- Natural flavorings
- Phytosphingosine extract
- Seasonings
- *Secale cereale*
- Soy protein
- Stabilizers
- Starch
- *Triticum aestivum*
- *Triticum vulgare*
- Vegetable protein
- Yeast extract

Gluten in Medicine and Over-the-Counter Products

Just when you think you are the expert on gluten-containing products and ingredients, there are even more products that might contain gluten that you must look out for. You have to be very diligent about what you purchase and consume with regards to supplements, vitamins, and medicines. Gluten ingredients are commonly used as binders, expedients, and coatings for pills (Gluten Free Gigi.com). Even over-the-counter medicines, vitamins, and supplements can contain gluten. Probiotics were even found to contain gluten. I check the label on any product that I consume to see if it is labeled as gluten-free, especially over-the-counter medicine. If not, I jump on my phone and call the manufacturer or check the Internet. Most large consumer product companies will quickly respond to calls regarding gluten-containing products. Otherwise, here is a great website to have on hand: http://www.glutenfreedrugs.com.

According to the website Gluten Free Gigi, "sometimes pharmaceutical companies don't know whether medicines contain gluten because they are unaware of how raw materials for their products are sourced or handled outside their facility" and "generic drugs may have different expedients (fillers and binders) than branded drugs." It's a good idea, if you're on long-term pharmaceuticals, to build a relationship with your pharmacist and have them contact you if a generic is being substituted so you can find the necessary information to make sure it is safe to consume.

You would never think that your lipstick or an envelope could bother your digestive system, but for some severe sufferers, these simple items can trigger a response. The following is a partial list of simple items that could cause a reaction:

- Pharmaceutical and over-the-counter drugs
- Cosmetics
- Dental hygienist cleaning products (toothpastes and latex gloves)
- Vitamins and supplements (cough drops, lozenges, etc.)
- Household cleaning products
- Stamps and envelopes
- Pet food
- Paints
- Play dough
- Suntan lotion
- Bath salts

FDA Labeling Laws

Gluten-free labeling was put into effect August of 2013. In order to label a product gluten-free, it must contain less than twenty parts per million of gluten-containing ingredients. Most commercial food products labeled as gluten-free still contain some gluten, although some contain less than others do. Foods that contain one part per million of gluten contain 0.0001 percent of gluten as a percentage of the food, while foods that contain twenty parts per million of gluten contain 0.002 percent gluten. That doesn't sound like a lot, but the more prepackaged food you eat, the more gluten you consume. Those parts per million can add up.

The FDA will allow manufacturers to label a food gluten-free if the food does **not** contain any of the following:

- An ingredient that is any type of wheat, rye, barley, or crossbreeds of these grains
- An ingredient derived from these grains that has been processed to remove gluten if it results in the food containing more than twenty parts per million of gluten

Foods, such as bottled spring water, fruits and vegetables, and eggs can also be labeled gluten-free if they inherently don't have any gluten.

FDA labeling does not apply to the following:

- USDA products
- Alcohol*
- Cosmetics
- Prescription drugs / nonprescription drugs
- Pet food

An important note about the twenty parts per million: **Testing to show twenty parts per million is not required; this is a voluntary statement.** People with celiac disease should still avoid anything containing barley malt or hydrolyzed wheat protein (US Food and Drug Administration). Always read the labels even if they are labeled gluten-free, and it never hurts to jump on the Internet to double-check ingredients as manufacturers will change ingredients and call it "new and improved" without reporting what has been changed.

*Avoid beer unless it is specifically brewed to be gluten-free. Wine is typically gluten-free along with most hard ciders. Rum, tequila, and potato vodka are gluten-free. Whiskey and bourbon are not universally accepted as gluten-free, so proceed with caution. (Gluten-Free Alcohol Guide)

Group Certifications

There are three organizations—the Gluten Intolerance Group's Gluten-Free Certification Organization (GFCO), the Celiac Sprue Association (CSA), and the National Foundation for Celiac Awareness (NFCA)—that currently certify products and companies as gluten-free. They are here to make our lives easier. No longer do we have to search through the ingredient list looking for hidden sources of gluten, or remember fancy names for gluten, these groups have done the work for us!

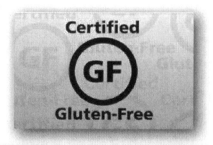

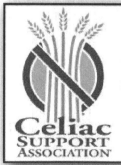

The appearance of this Seal on packaging certifies: (1) that the manufacturer adheres to the Celiac Support Association® (CSA) standards – free of wheat, barley, rye, and common oats, their crosses and derivatives in product, processing and packaging; or (2) that innovative products have been crafted to remove the gluten from the finished product.

Verification testing must confirm no detectable gluten using the most appropriate analysis for the product.

Visit CSA at www.csaceliacs.org or call toll-free 877-CSA-4-CSA.

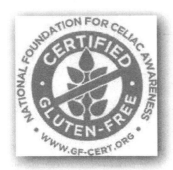

These certification programs have various standards and test for different levels of trace gluten in the foods they certify. The Gluten-Free Certification Organization, for example, tests foods to make sure they contain less than ten parts per million of gluten. The National Foundation for Celiac Awareness program also tests foods to ten parts per million. The Celiac Sprue Association, meanwhile, requires foods to have less than five parts per million, a more stringent standard, and requires foods to be free of oats (even gluten-free oats).

Another great resource is The Celiac Foundation. They sponsor gluten-free events, raise money for awareness, and their website is packed with information. They have a listing for local support groups as well.

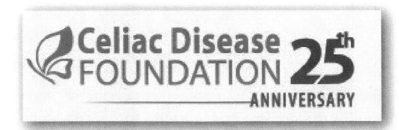

All of these organizations are not-for-profit so giving to them financially will help to ensure they will be able to continue providing this important information.

National Foundation for Celiac Awareness
http://www.celiaccentral.org/SiteData/d/NFCA_mail_donation.pdf

Gluten Intolerance Group
https://www.gluten.net/donate/

Celiac Sprue
https://www.csaceliacs.org/donate_now.jsp

Celiac Disease Foundation
http://celiac.org/get-involved/donate-2/

Step 2

Transition

Have a Good (Great) Attitude

The first thing you need to say to yourself after being diagnosed with a gluten intolerance is,

"This is a blessing, not a curse."

That will set the tone for the rest of your life. It's hard to have the food you love taken away. Food for me was the memories of my childhood, traditions during the holidays, and comfort through life. Nothing makes you feel better when you are sick or sad like your mom's soup or a warm piece of toast and some tea. After I was diagnosed with gluten intolerance, I took on the mantra that "this *is* a blessing." Once I transitioned over and started to feel better I knew it was time to stop making excuses for the positive way I was eating when people questioned why I was eating gluten-free.

It's okay to mourn what you have lost, such as the flavors, textures, and memories food brought to you. But, don't let it control your life. You know you are angry about your situation when you spend the whole day with what my celiac brother-in-law calls "carb entitlement." He says that he is allowed to eat a lot of other carbohydrates because his favorite carbs have been taken away (mostly his mom's homemade pies, cakes, and sweets). When your thoughts on what everyone else is eating around you begin to consume you, it's time to tell yourself, "This is happening *for* me, not *to* me!"

It's important to keep balance in your life. Losing gluten doesn't give you a license to go out and eat every other unhealthy grain product on the market, but it also shouldn't be a reason to give up eating things you enjoy. You just need to find your balance, learn how to make the transition, and start looking at your whole attitude about food and nutrition to make changes where necessary.

Take a moment to write down three things that are going well in your life right now despite the fact you have a gluten intolerance. For example, your diagnosis now enables you take action to finally feel better. That is reason to celebrate and to be thankful.

Write three things going well in your life now:

1.

2.

3.

Find New Foods to Love and to Make

Be positive. That was what I needed to tell myself. I was determined that it was no longer going to be about what foods I had to eliminate, but about what new foods I could find or what new ingredients I could substitute. It wasn't going to be about what I lost, but instead about what I found new to eat or to make.

The first twelve months after going gluten-free were difficult to say the least. There were only a few gluten-free items on the shelves, so I couldn't find substitutes for foods easily. I spent a lot of time and money trying to replace the flavors and textures I lost in my gluten-full foods. Nothing tasted the same, so I had to change my thought process, and rather than mourn what I lost, I had to find new foods to love or new ways to make them. Instead of birthday cake, my husband would get me mango-flavored water ice from Rita's Water Ice. My kids loved it, and it became a new way to celebrate in my home.

Another way to find new foods is to explore foods from other countries. For example, we eat a lot of Mexican food now since it uses a lot of corn-based products (corn tortillas and chips). Fresh, homemade salsa and guacamole are a family favorite. Japanese sushi is always fun because of the many choices and textures available (but remember to substitute the soy sauce with tamari). I've even gotten my family to try different combinations for fish and vegetables by learning to make sushi at home. It's amazing what kids will try when it's something they make themselves.

Open your heart and mind to trying new textures and flavors, and you will be surprised what new gluten-free foods you will enjoy.

Here's a great exercise to open your heart and mind to new foods:

List three gluten-full foods you lost

1.

2.

3.

List three new gluten-free foods you found

1.

2.

3.

Old Traditions with New Flavors and Ingredients

Holidays are huge in my family. As the baby (aka Bebe) of ten children (seven girls and three boys) in a very traditional Eastern European, Slovak/Ukrainian home, food was a big part of each holiday. My mother made sure that we enjoyed all the foods that she (and my Ukrainian dad) had as children during the holidays. Pierogis and mushroom soup at Christmas and ham and nut rolls at Easter were just a few of the foods that were connected to each holiday. Going gluten-free was just as traumatic for my family (as it was for me) to keep me connected to our family traditions while trying not to make me sick. My mother, who was eighty-one at the time, said, "What am I going to do about you?"

When it was time to cook dinner she didn't want to leave anyone out, so she had to adapt old recipes to be gluten-free without making the whole family upset. I found gluten-free frozen pierogis and my sister Sue made the Christmas mushroom soup gluten-free and dairy-free, and no one knew the difference. Another sister even made her family's traditional Italian wedding soup with gluten-free chicken stock and noodles for us to enjoy.

In the four years I have been gluten-free, there are many more convenient ingredients available for substitutes. There are flours that can be substituted cup for cup into old recipes, which makes baking so much easier. Xanthan gum (the replacement for gluten) is already included into the flour blends, so there is no need to add them separately. (See gluten-free flour blends in the "Substitution" section of the book.)

A great thing to do around the holidays is to write down your favorite recipes (as you think of them) and circle the ingredients that might contain gluten and will need a substitution. Try the new ingredients with the old recipes and keep notes each year until the flavors become more familiar to what you remember. It took my sister two years, but she finally perfected her gluten-free and dairy-free nut rolls. She took notes the last two Christmases on texture and flavor, and even wrote a couple notes on what to try next year. Sure enough, this year, her nut rolls had the perfect taste and texture! It might be a challenge at first, but recognizing gluten-containing ingredients is a great skill to learn as you transition into a gluten-free lifestyle.

To get you started, write down some holiday foods that you love. What might need to be substituted to make them gluten-free?

Holiday	Food	Gluten-Free Substitution
Example: Christmas	Russian Tea Cake Cookies	Gluten-free flour blend
		Gluten-free powdered sugar

Don't Depend on Prepackaged Gluten-Free Foods

It's always tempting to fill your cabinets with quick, easy to grab food items. I'm guilty of it. As a matter of fact, the third section of this book ("Substitution") is all about what prepackaged products can be substituted back into your pantry to make your life easier. We are all part of a society that is used to having everything fast and easy, so when you are hungry, you just want to reach into your pantry and satiate your needs immediately. The problem with doing that while on a gluten-free diet is that although food is our body's medicine, it sometimes costs as much as our medicines. For example, a fourteen-ounce bag of gluten-free pretzels is $6.99 versus $2.98 for a sixteen-ounce bag of gluten-full. I found that a four-ounce pack of gluten-free crackers is $4.99 versus sixteen ounces of gluten-full crackers for $3.80. As a matter of fact, the average gluten-free food product is 242 percent more expensive than the gluten-full version. Gluten-free sales will be more than $5 billion in 2015, so someone is making good money on gluten-free!

Walking into your food pantry can be a depressing thing if you don't have quick things to eat, especially when you are hungry. A good way to think about gluten-free prepackaged foods is that they are a vehicle to get something naturally gluten-free into your mouth. Gluten-free crackers or pretzels are handy to get nut butters, hummus, or cheese into your system. At the end of the book, I include a great recipe for hummus to enjoy.

Although most potato chips are gluten-free, it's not a license to eat the entire bag. Portion control is so important with gluten-free foods, because most prepackaged gluten-free products contain one-third more calories, sugar and sodium and less fiber. It's no surprise that the average person gains twenty-two pounds on a gluten-free diet. Granted, most people are nutritionally deficient before going gluten-free, but prepackaged gluten-free foods are not fortified like gluten-full products, so it really doesn't help increase those nutrients. For example, gluten-free breads don't get the niacin, riboflavin, and iron that the gluten-full grain products are fortified with, so eating more gluten-free products won't give you the nutrients that your body needs.

A very important thing to keep in mind is that gluten-free products are often made with high glycemic grains, like white rice, corn, and potato that raise blood sugar and insulin levels in the body quickly. Learning to substitute lower glycemic alternative grains, such as quinoa, buckwheat, or amaranth, is key to eating a healthier gluten-free diet. Eating these whole grains will not only increase nutrient content, they will bring costs down too.

Naturally gluten-free foods are always easy to grab as well. Fruits, vegetables, meats, cheeses, and nuts are naturally gluten-free. Eating things in the whole form are also safer to eat with regards to cross contamination (we'll talk more about that later).

Here are the key things to remember about gluten-free prepackaged foods:

- Can contain up to one-third more calories
- Higher in sodium
- Not fortified
- Made with higher glycemic grains (corn and rice)
- Cost more
- One-quarter more carbs
- More sugar

Always Be Prepared

This is a hard lesson to learn, but the quicker you realize that eating gluten-free safely is *your* challenge, the less heartache and terrible experiences of being "glutened" you will have. There is always disappointment when you go somewhere unprepared and there is nothing safe for you to eat. A perfect example of this is driving on the Pennsylvania turnpike. If you have ever stopped at one of the rest areas along this expansive road, you would see that there is very little for a gluten-free person to eat. I'm not talking high-quality food, just any gluten-free food. Pizza, burgers, fried foods, and pretzels along with every other type of fast food, but almost nothing for the gluten-sensitive community. It can be a depressing place if you aren't prepared and you are hungry. This is where I learned that it's my responsibility to bring foods that are safe for me to eat—*all* the time!

I make sure I make a meal, carry a Power Bar, some nuts, and have some fruits and vegetables available every time I get in the car. You can never be too prepared. I eliminated the idea that every company is going to provide safe food for me to eat, and that I can't risk eating food that *might* be okay. This is when prepackaged gluten-free foods can come in handy. A bag of gluten-free pretzels can be a savior, so paying seven dollars for a bag is worth it on a four-hour car ride from Philadelphia to Pittsburgh, Pennsylvania.

I like to take the pressure off my friends too. When I'm invited to someone's house, I always bring my own gluten-free beverage as well as some chips and dip to share. If you bring it, you know you can eat it. My advice is don't even bother telling your friend you are bringing something, just walk into the house carrying a hot dip or a giant container of Chex Mix for everyone to share. Everyone will devour it, and you will too.

Here is a list of snacks to take on a car trip to be prepared:

- Individual packs of nut butters (almond, peanut butter, cashew, sun butter, etc.)
- Hummus and chips
- Cut-up fruits and vegetables (clementine oranges are a hit in our car!)
- Nut/protein bars (see the end of the book for a homemade nut bar recipe)
- Meat (turkey jerky, dried meat sticks, pepperoni, salami, or other gluten-free lunch meat, rolled)
- Cheese sticks or cubes
- Nuts
- Gluten-free pretzels
- Homemade Chex Mix
- Homemade granola
- Gluten-free salad dressing and soy sauce packets
- A good piece of chocolate

Notes about traveling snacks:

Safe Restaurant Eating

There have been periods over the last few years that I boy-cotted eating out after repeatedly being glutened by res-taurants. I swear 90 percent of my glutening experiences happen after eating at a fast food restaurant. I don't make a habit of taking my kids to eat fast food, but sometimes you've got to do what you've got to do and are forced to eat at one. I would just tell myself, "Yes, you are probably going to get sick after eating this."

It's important to remember that fast food restaurants aren't the best choices for gluten-free options, but it's not necessarily their fault. Most (not all) don't have a designated gluten-free prep area to work in, so the risk of cross con-tamination is much higher in that fast-paced environment. The choice of fast food restaurants usually comes on quickly (with hunger), so it's always helpful to do an Internet search of your children's favorite places to see what is listed on their websites as safe before you decide to eat there. Some restaurants have published menus, so keeping a copy of them in your car's glove box with gluten-free items circled is an easy way to stay safe while on the road. When I'm trav-eling, I look for Wendy's. Their baked potato and chili are both gluten-free. Chick-fil-A has several items listed on their website as "not containing gluten ingredients." Specifically, their french fries, grilled chicken nuggets, and several salads.

It's good to know what's available locally to eat. We have several family owned restaurants in the area that have a gluten-free menu. I know the owners personally, and I trust what they are serving is safe, so I give them my business. In return for their gluten-free menu choices, I tell everyone to eat there. It's a win-win for the owners and me. If they stay in business, I have a safe place to go out to eat. Our local family restaurant Liberty Union had their staff trained by the Gluten Intolerance Group (GIG), and their kitchen is now certified by their organization, so it's a no-brainer to eat there.

Talking to other gluten-intolerant friends about where they eat is always helpful. I find new places to eat every time I talk to my celiac friend Jill. She is a wealth of information and is always happy to tell friends about her new culinary finds. She introduced me to a great app called Find Me Gluten Free (www.findmeglutenfree.com). Just pop that app on your phone, and it automatically locates all the safe restaurants in your vicinity. Another great website to use when you are looking for someplace to eat is www.celiactravel.com. Or you can search for gluten-free restaurants in your area using www.opentable.com.

It's my experience that larger corporate restaurants seem (in most cases) to be good about gluten-free food preparation. Although they usually have an "eat at your own risk" explanation about not being able to prevent cross contamination, I find if the server is gluten-free savvy, he or she was probably trained that way. If a server doesn't have a clue about food sensitivities or has to call a manager over, be cautious. Chipotle is a great example of good employee training. They will change their gloves and follow you through the ordering process if you tell them it's for a food allergy, no questions asked.

Calling ahead and talking to the manager or even the chef is a great way to get information and relieve the stress of eating out. Last summer I attended my friend's wedding. It was a fabulous Latin affair with tons of great food. I was thrilled when I called the venue the day before and my friend already arranged to have something safe prepared for me for dinner. I was overwhelmed that the wait staff was already aware of it. How nice was that?

The website Gluten-Free Guide HQ (http://glutenfree-guidehq.com/chain-restaurants/) has an extensive list of chain restaurants that have gluten-free menus available.

Checklist of what to do before eating out:

- Look at the menu online.
- Make reservations using **www.opentable.com**, and search gluten-free-friendly restaurants. You can even send a message to the establishment asking for gluten-free menu items.
- Call ahead and talk to the manager or chef about what they recommend on their menu.
- Have a smartphone handy to search **www.find-meglutenfree.com** and download the app.
- Search fast food restaurants and know what you can eat before you pull in.
- Have these websites available: **www.celiactravel.com**, **http://www.qsrmagazine.com/news/allerg-yeats-releases-2014-list-allergy-friendly-chains.**
- Consult **http://glutenfreeguidehq.com/chain-restaurants/** to find which chains have gluten-free menu items.

Notes on eating out:

Know Your Resources

Your most important place to start, is your health care professional. You need to build a relationship with your doctor, nutritionist, and his or her office staff. Through proper testing, they can help you understand what your body looks like on the inside, how much damage you may have, and what additional tools you may need to heal it. You need to have a health care professional as an advocate for your health. Getting to know the office can also open doors to information—new drugs, treatments, articles, and suggestions on what to do if you get glutened. Also connect with your local hospital and see if they offer any gluten health-related seminars. My local hospital sends out a monthly e-mail showing the topics for talks on nutrition and health available to attend. Most are sponsored by the same doctors that diagnose gluten sensitivities, so you may see your own doctor at one of the events.

Western medicine practices are great, but I am a firm believer in also finding an Eastern medicine practitioner, a naturopathic doctor (ND), or a holistic practitioner to support you as well. It's a yin and yang approach to health. An Eastern or holistic professional will provide you an additional view to the Western philosophies and science.

Health coaches trained in nutrition are another great resource to seek out. They are also trained to provide emotional support, help you set reasonable health goals, and give suggestions on positive wellness practices. Other types of health care professionals are not trained to offer the emotional support that health coaches do, so the coaches are a great addition to your resource list. You can find a health coach through the American Association of Drugless Practioners (AADP) website at http://www.aadp. net. You can even become a health coach through the Institute for Integrative Nutrition (IIN) like I did. Their web-site is http://www.integrativenutrition.com/.

You are not alone in the gluten-free world. Many peo-ple have paved the way for the gluten-free community, and they want to pass information on to you. Finding those people (and organizations) and making those connections is easy with social media. Facebook and the Internet are good places to start.

For gluten-related information, the Internet is a key resource. Look for blogs (such as www.glutenfreebebe. com), websites, support groups, and organizations to pro-vide helpful information. Just search the word *gluten* and you will find 142 million places to look for information! With that, two of the best resources for information I found are the Gluten Intolerance Group (GIG) and the National Foundation for Celiac Awareness (NFCA).

GIG provides small group networking with quarterly meetings at various locations. I have attended many GIG sponsored talks and speaking programs, and it's amazing how many wonderful people you meet that are fighting the same battles as you. Our local chapter has fun dinners at gluten-safe restaurants, restaurant tours, product reviews, coupons, and bulk buying opportunities. It's a great organization to be an active member of.

The NFCA is a local, not-for-profit organization that provides information and brings public awareness about gluten-related disorders. Their website is packed with free pamphlets, webinars, and other resources and how tos on navigating gluten sensitivities inside and outside the home. They are a huge advocate for the FDA labeling laws and continue to fight (legislatively) for safe manufacturing practices for gluten-related products.

Finally, read, read, read. In addition to doing Internet searches, subscribe to magazines, find books at the library, and search Facebook, Twitter, and Pinterest. Don't stop learning, asking questions, and searching. Just make sure the information is from credible sources. The more you read about gluten intolerance, the easier it is to understand it and to adopt treatments into your daily routine.

Here is a list of resources:

- **Gluten Intolerance Group (GIG): https://www.gluten.net/**
- **National Foundation for Celiac Awareness (NFCA): http://www.celiaccentral.org/**
- **Celiac Sprue: http://www.csaceliacs.org/**
- **Celiac Disease Foundation: http://celiac.org/**

- **American Association of Drugless Practitioners: http://www.aadp.net/**
- **Functional Medicine Doctors: http://www.func-tionalmedicinedoctors.com/**
- **Gluten-Free Bebe: http://www.glutenfreebebe. com** My website, blog and Facebook pages are filled with gluten-free and nutritional information.

A Message to Your Family

Having a gluten sensitivity (of any degree) is traumatic for the sufferer, but what about the family members? I'm talking about the moms, dads, sisters, brothers, husbands, children, extended family, friends, etc. of the gluten-sensitive person. It's easy to get frustrated when eating out or to get melancholy when new ingredients need to get introduced to old recipes, but it's important that you keep positive, so your gluten-free family member can keep positive as well.

Celiac disease affects about three million Americans and gluten sensitivity significantly more, although the majority of them are not diagnosed. That's a lot of people, and chances are, you are going to run across someone else with a gluten intolerance that you might be able to offer encouragement (or kindness and empathy) to in your lifetime.

Gluten-intolerance sufferers worry about food and the difficulty of finding safe food a lot. If you are a family member of a gluten-intolerant sufferer, here are some things to remember:

- Be supportive and encouraging. It can be a difficult transition to gluten-free living.
- Be empathetic. Being glutened and feeling sick is no fun.

- Be patient, especially when preparing new food or when eating out.
- Be an advocate. Try to make yourself knowledge-able about gluten intolerance.
- Be open minded. Begin to explore holistic health and be supportive of it. Remember food is medicine!

Talking to Your Family about Celiac Testing

As I have experienced with my own family, talking about celiac can be very difficult. I'm very passionate about the subject and I'm always concerned about other family members suffering from gluten-related symptoms. I've tried to encourage other family members to be tested for celiac, but it's difficult to convince family that it's necessary without sounding like a nag.

There are lots of dos and don'ts to remember when bringing up the subject for the first time. It is a hereditary disease, so the best way to start a conversation is to be very factual (see facts that follow). If you are gluten intolerant, I recommend you also talk about your own experiences in addition to the higher risks of certain diseases associated with celiac (certain cancers, autoimmune thyroiditis, type I diabetes). Try to bring up the subject face to face, and share educational material. Don't use e-mail or social media as it may become combative if too many people get involved at the same time. Finally, don't focus on the diet as that will discourage them from getting tested. If you need more information on how to talk to your family about testing, the NFCA (http://www.celiaccentral.org/talktelltest/) offers great resources on their website about the subject.

Here are some interesting facts about celiac disease:

- One in one hundred thirty-three Americans have celiac disease, but 95 percent remain undiagnosed.
- Three million Americans have celiac, but only 150,000 know they have it.
- One in twenty-two celiac patients have a close relative (parent, child, sibling) with celiac.
- It takes an average of four years to get diagnosed with celiac.
- Sixty percent of children and 41 percent of adults diagnosed were without any symptoms.
- Only 35 percent of newly diagnosed patients had chronic diarrhea.
- Only 25 percent of celiac cases present with any gastrointestinal symptoms.
- If diagnosed with celiac from two to four years of age, there is a 10.5 percent chance of developing a second autoimmune disorder.
- One-thirtieth of a slice of bread can cause mucosal inflammation in a celiac.
- One sixty-fourth of a teaspoon of gluten can cause intestinal damage in a celiac.
- Celiac can show up at any time or any age, so it's a good idea to get tested every two to three years if there is a family member that is already diagnosed.

Challenges of Being Gluten-Free in a Gluten-Full House

Let me start by saying I could write an entire book on this topic alone because I'm living this every day in my home. Looking back to when I made the decision to go gluten-free, I wanted everyone in my house to eat gluten-free with me. I bought all new gluten-free cereals, healthy snacks, and eliminated sugary foods as much as I could. Boy was I wrong! Too much too fast was very hard for my children. Although I could see that they would benefit from a gluten-free diet, I forgot how traumatic it was for me, let alone them. I forgot to remind myself that I had survived on a gluten-full diet for forty-plus years (not too well, but I did survive).

They were just getting used to the fact that Mom couldn't eat familiar things, and I wanted to take their comfort foods away too. My son said it perfectly, "This gluten-free organic thing is pulling our family apart." So much of eating is peer related, and children need to eat what their peers eat. I had to reevaluate what I was buying and find balance.

I decided to divide the family and make it a gluten-free and gluten-full house, until I could get a good grasp on what products were available for everyone to eat. The biggest challenge after making the decision to be a house divided was preventing cross contamination. It only takes one-eighth teaspoon of flour (one-half crouton) to cause an autoimmune response in a celiac patient, so organizing my food pantry was a primary goal. I took all the gluten-free products and placed them on a shelf high up in the food pantry. They were placed high for two reasons. One, so that gluten-full crumbs and dust couldn't fall on them from above and two, they are expensive. It never fails, when you pay more for something, everyone wants it. I had to hide my gluten-free cookies and snacks so that when I wanted them, there was still some to eat. I even put items on the gluten-free shelf that were naturally gluten-free, like quinoa, rice, and instant mashed potatoes. That way I knew what pantry items were available as ingredients for other recipes as well.

Although I decided to divide the house into gluten-free/gluten-full with regards to snacks, I also decided to make all dinners gluten-free. For a period, I made my portions separate, but it just made more sense to make recipes that were naturally gluten-free or that contained ingredients that everyone could enjoy. For example, I don't make separate pasta for myself; everyone eats gluten-free noodles. My children didn't really notice that change, but my husband did. Thankfully, he was willing to eat the pasta he was given to make my life easier. I use gluten-free breading (e.g., gluten-free panko) for recipes, and I thicken soups and gravies with rice flour or cornstarch. What you don't tell them, they won't know, so be choosy about what ingredient information you share.

Some gluten-free pantry items are expensive and come in smaller portions. The average gluten-free product is 242 percent more expensive than the regular version. So planning your meals is helpful. I look at old recipes and try to change ingredients with something already in my pantry. For example, if a recipe calls for canned soups (which usually contain gluten), I might use dried or fresh herbs, fresh vegetables, and chicken stock, and I use instant mashed potatoes to thicken. It's a lot less expensive than buying a bunch of gluten-free soups that no one but me can eat.

Another area that needs to be gluten-free is the refrigerator. Keeping a shelf on the door for safe condiments or marking the safe foods with a special sticker or colored tape will alert everyone that these items are for special recipes. It's also helpful when the kids can help themselves to the items that are clearly marked as safe. It cuts down on having everyone ask Mom, "Can you eat this?"

Kitchen equipment, including flatware, serving utensils, baking sheets, cutting boards, strainers, toasters, and pans are also hidden sources for cross contamination. Just take a look at all the crumbs in the bottom of your flatware or utensil drawer. Those crumbs add up quickly. Remember one-eighth teaspoon of flour can cause an autoimmune response.

Duplicate medicines, cleaning supplies, makeup, and personal products might be necessary.

Key takeaways about a gluten-free/gluten-full house are

- Keep gluten-free pantry products up high on their own shelf.
- Keep a refrigerator door shelf for gluten-free products.
- Clean the utensil drawer often.
- Color code utensils, colanders, and cutting boards.
- Consider buying separate pots and pans, toaster, and strainer.
- Label a separate container for safe gluten-free medicines.

Step 3

Substitution

Thoughts about Nutrition

Becoming gluten-free is a perfect time to change bad food and nutrition habits. By adopting more whole, naturally gluten-free fresh foods, you can ease yourself into the gluten-free lifestyle. Fruits, vegetables, organic meats, and cheeses are all gluten-free, so they take the fear out of eating. You constantly have to tell yourself that eating gluten-free is *not* a diet. It can be very healthy like a new diet, but it's medically necessary, so consider it your medicine rather than a fad diet. You wouldn't want to choose one gluten-free food to eat for weeks like you might on a weight loss program. We've all heard of the grapefruit diet or the cabbage soup diet, which are all gluten-free, but are not the nutritionally well-rounded way of eating long term. If you constantly remind yourself that this is your medicine, then making choices about what needs to be substituted back into your pantry will be easier.

The average person gains twenty-two pounds on a gluten-free diet. This is mostly because the people who eat gluten-free are nutritionally deficient and haven't been absorbing any of the nutrients they are consuming. However, a lot of the weight is from the high amounts of sugar and carbohydrates that prepackaged gluten-free foods contain (one-third more calories, one-quarter more carbs, and lower in fiber). People who find relief from a gluten-free lifestyle feel better because something toxic has been removed from their diet. Don't choose to eliminate one type of toxin (gluten) from your body, only to choose a different one (i.e., sugar, saturated fat) to add back in. *If you eat a box of cookies, gluten-free or not, you will gain weight!*

One way to look at your food pantry is to say to yourself, "What do I need in my pantry as a vehicle to get something fresh, locally produced, and naturally gluten-free into my system?" For example, a gluten-free cracker is perfect to get some handcrafted, locally made cheese into your body. Or, look at your chip as a vehicle to scoop some fresh homemade salsa.

This section is all about what products are available from the grocery store that I have found to be good substitutions for gluten-containing products. This chapter separates me from other health coaches. My health coach training tells me that I should be encouraging you to not buy any prepackaged products (gluten-free or not). The reality is, the quicker you become compliant with a gluten-free diet, the quicker you will feel better. So, if you need to buy a gluten-free cake mix to keep you from cheating and eating a piece of gluten-full cake at a birthday party, then buy the gluten-free brand, make it, share it, and stay gluten-free without the urge to cheat.

As we all know, when you are hungry, it's sometimes difficult to concentrate and think of what might be healthy to eat quickly. Here are ten quick and healthy snacks to grab when the urge arises:

- Nut butter with gluten-free pretzels or apples
- Celery with Laughing Cow cheese
- Fruit smoothies
- Hummus with veggies or gluten-free chips
- Yogurt with nuts, seeds, and/or fruit
- Nuts
- Edamame
- Fruit with cheese
- Popcorn
- Chips and salsa
- Homemade kale chips
- Olives

Eat Fresh and Local

Eating fresh ingredients is a perfect way to get nutrients into your body. Most gluten-intolerant sufferers have some sort of intestinal damage (leaky gut) from years of eating the wrong foods. In order to help your gut heal, you not only have to eliminate gluten, but also you need to choose foods that will build and strengthen your immune system. Choosing high nutrient content foods, like locally grown, organic produce, is a great way to help your body heal.

Because nutrient content goes down as soon as fresh foods are picked, the closer to home the food is grown, the more nutrients it will have. This is true for not only fruits and vegetables but also meat, poultry, and dairy products, which have more nutrients than industrial farmed animal products (Klavinski).

Local ingredients produce more flavorful foods. Fresh picked ingredients are usually placed in stores within twenty four hours. This means farmers try to pick produce at the peak of freshness. Compare that to foods picked on the other side of the earth and shipped to your local stores. It may take days or weeks to get from the farm to the table if it's produced on another continent. Think about that the next time you are eating blueberries from Chile in December.

Supporting the local farmer is good for everyone. Keeping money and jobs close to home helps preserve farms, open space, and families in our communities. A good place to start when looking for local farm markets, farm stands, or community-supported agriculture (CSA) farms is on the Internet. The website Local Harvest allows you to enter in your zip code to find farms, farm stands, and CSAs in your area: http://www.localharvest.org/csa/.

In Pennsylvania, you can go to http://www.pafarm.com to find farms to purchase from. Another organization that brings farmers together is the Pennsylvania Association for Sustainable Agriculture (PASA). They always have programs to teach farmers how to connect with consumers. Many large universities offer information about local farming. For example, Penn State University has a searchable function on their website to find a CSA in your area: http://extension.psu.edu/business/farm/csa. Finally, http://www.buylocalpa.org/ provides all kinds of information on local products. Pennsylvania is lucky to have lots of resources for consumers to connect with farmers, so check the Internet for a similar organization in your area.

One of my favorite things to do in the summer is preserve local foods to enjoy all year by hot-water canning or freezing items. For example, canned (or frozen) tomatoes, corn, and beans can be added to soups or roasts in the winter. Instead of eating blueberries from Chile in December, why not freeze some local berries and enjoy a fruit cobbler as a treat? See my recipe section for a great tomato and cobbler recipe.

Notes about fresh and local products:

Go Organic

I have many friends that roll their eyes over the subject of organic versus conventional foods. I know organic products are more expensive, and nutritionally they are no different from conventional foods, but buy organic to help your gut heal. By definition, organic farming is a "form of agriculture that relies on techniques such as crop rotation, green manure, compost, and biological pest control." According to Wikipedia, organic farming "uses fertilizers and pesticides (which include herbicides, insecticides, and fungicides) if they are considered natural (such as bone meal from animals or pyrethrin from flowers), but it excludes or strictly limits the use of various methods (including synthetic petrochemical fertilizers and pesticides; plant growth regulators such as hormones; antibiotic use in livestock; genetically modified organisms) for reasons including sustainability, openness, independence, health, and safety." (Wikipedia, "Organic Farming," 2015)

The whole reason eating gluten-free helps people is that it allows damage in their intestines to heal. By eating organic and not consuming pesticides in your foods, you can begin to absorb the nutrients your foods have to offer. Most gluten-intolerant sufferers are deficient in many nutrients (iron, B vitamins, ferritin, and calcium, just to name a few), so choose to consume high-quality foods that naturally contain the nutrients your body needs without pesticides. Eating organic, whenever possible, is a great way to help the environment as well. Less pesticides and fungicides means less run off into our water and richer, more nutrient-dense soil too.

It sounds hard, but it's not. For every prepackaged food, eat a fresh organically produced food with it. Wondering where to find organic fresh foods? Find a local farm market, join a CSA, or make friends with a farmer and find out where he or she shops. Choose organic when you can. Sometimes quality is better than quantity, so buying a few things from the dirty dozen list, which follows, is better than choosing none.

- Apples
- Strawberries
- Grapes
- Celery
- Peaches
- Spinach
- Sweet bell peppers
- Nectarines (imported)
- Cucumbers
- Cherry tomatoes
- Snap peas (imported)
- Potatoes

Eat Seasonally

Eating seasonally is another smart way to choose gluten-free foods. Eating foods that support you during each of the four seasons will help strengthen your immune system naturally. For example, eat foods to hydrate your body during the heat of summer, like watermelon. Or eat vitamin D-rich foods like mushrooms and dark greens in the winter when there is less sun exposure. A bowl of beef broth in the winter will naturally give your body the calcium it needs, whereas in the spring, when you don't need heavy fats, lighter greens help detox the liver and gallbladder from its long sleepy winter.

When you think about it, it just makes sense. We *can* eat certain foods all year long, but *should* we? Our bodies were designed to protect us during different seasons, so to eat foods out of season can overload our systems, which may be the cause for so many food intolerances. Rotating foods in our diets keeps our body balanced, thus preventing imbalances and/or intolerances (Luisa).

For example, eating lots of fats in the winter helps us stay warm. In Chinese medicine, spring's bounty helps to cleanse the liver of all its winter toxins. By eating cleansing foods at the wrong time, our liver gets off balance and that can upset our systems.

Each time I eat a peach in December, I think about what that fruit went through to get to me in Pennsylvania. Industrialized farming has to bend nature's rules in order for the food to survive improper seasons (Luisa). Perhaps the fruit or vegetable was picked before its peak, so the nutrients aren't fully developed. It then may be subjected to gas (ethylene) to force ripeness and make it look more presentable on the store's shelf.

Here are some suggestions on what GF foods to eat during different seasons:

Summer:
- Foods that provide adequate liquids to stay hydrated (tomatoes, melons)
- Fruits and vegetables (watermelon, cucumbers, strawberries)
- Lean proteins (chicken and fish)

Fall:
- Foods that help prepare our bodies for winter and add moisture
- Nuts, seeds, onion, ginger, peppers, apples, pears, grapefruits, lemon, pineapple, honey, dairy products

Winter:
- Foods to conserve energy and add warmth
- Beef, eggs, mushroom, kale, root vegetables
- Reduce salt intake

Spring:

- Food to help cleanse the liver and protect the body against flu
- Fresh green and leafy vegetables, bananas, pears, celery
- Avoid greasy foods to protect the spleen and build immune system

Choose Alternative Grains

The first week of going gluten-free, I walked into my pantry. I was hungry and needed something to eat immediately, and a rice cake was not going to do it. I ate potato chips night and day. Potatoes, rice, and corn were the three quick and safe ingredients I could think of to eat when hunger erupted. Unfortunately, none of them helped my underlying digestive issues. They are all high-glycemic grains, so as soon as I ate them, I was hungry again and of course ate more. Most of the prepackaged products were covered in salt, and none of the products helped me lose any weight.

It wasn't until I started to explore alternative grains such as brown rice, quinoa, buckwheat, teff, and amaranth that I could satiate my hunger. Eating these grains in their "whole" form is also better for you. I started to toast quinoa and add it to my granola. I popped organic popcorn and had it for a snack in the afternoon or enjoyed gluten-free oats for breakfast.

Gluten-free prepackaged foods are not required to be fortified, so many products don't provide additional nutrients and minerals that are added to their gluten-full counterparts. For example, products containing wheat (like bread) have been fortified with extra vitamins and nutrients like niacin, iron, and calcium to help prevent malnutrition. By choosing naturally gluten-free grains that are higher in certain micronutrients, however, you can help your body heal from malnutrition caused by gluten digestive problems.

Here is a list of gluten-free whole grain options:

- Buckwheat (high in fiber, B vitamins, and iron)
- Millet (magnesium, niacin)
- Quinoa (high protein, fiber, B vitamins, iron, and amino acids)
- Teff (thiamin, B6)
- Amaranth (calcium, iron, and fiber)
- Brown rice (magnesium and selenium)
- Sorghum (fiber and iron)

Treat Yourself Like Royalty

What does this have to do with being gluten-free? So much of eating gluten-free is about healing the damaging effects of gluten in the body. Food quality is more important than quantity, especially with gluten-damaged systems. We all agree that "we are what we eat." Literally the apple we consume helps to become our skin, hair, and nails, so why not eat the highest-quality apple available? Seventy percent of our immune system is in our digestive organs, so putting high-quality foods into our bodies helps build a stronger immune system from the inside out.

Now, I don't think denying yourself every sugary food you love is the most realistic thing to do. Instead, treat yourself like a queen or king. Choose only sweets that would be worthy of you. A high-quality piece of dark chocolate is much more enjoyable, and perhaps provides more antioxidants, than a candy bar from a gas station convenience store. Sometimes less is more, so enjoy the finer things that life has to offer.

Remember quality versus quantity!

Cook at Home More Often

The first year of being gluten-free, it didn't feel like it was making a difference in my life. After much trial and error, I finally realized that in order to feel better, I had to eliminate gluten and give my gut the opportunity to heal. Ingesting a little gluten here and there added up, and it would not allow me to feel well. For example, I would feel great Tuesday through Friday, eat out on Friday, and feel awful on Monday. It was a terrible cycle. It finally dawned on me what the likely cause was: what I ate at the end of one week would affect me at the beginning of the next. Although I was not choosing gluten-containing food, I was inadvertently being glutened by the restaurants.

Once I figured that out, I decided to eat at home as often as I could to allow my digestive system to heal. Once the inflammation went down and I was feeling better, I would try to see how long I could go without being glutened again. When I felt bad, I could always count back three days to a restaurant I had eaten at.

The hardest thing for me to figure out was why I continued to have migraines on Wednesdays sometimes. I thought I was always very careful about what I ate, but there were still Wednesdays that I felt ill even when I had not eaten out over the weekend. It finally dawned on me that it was the communion host I was receiving each Sunday at my church! At that time I had no idea that one-quarter of a communion host was all it took to cause an autoimmune response. Lucky for me, our parish now offers a low-gluten host, which allows me to participate in services without feeling ill on Wednesdays.

Everyone has varying degrees of sensitivities, but unless you eliminate gluten 100 percent, you will never know how much you can tolerate. Don't think that you will *never get to* eat out again, but just give your body the chance to heal and get strong before you venture out into the gluten-full world.

Trying to eat at home every night can be a huge adjustment, so learn to cook once and eat twice, meaning that you make enough food for two days' worth of meals. That cuts down cooking to only three to four times a week, instead of seven different meals.

For example, cook enough plain pasta for two meals. Serve a red sauce one night and vegetable primavera another night. When you roast the vegetables for the pasta, cook extra and blend some with chicken stock to make soup for a second meal. You need to be a bit creative, but you can do it with a little planning.

Here's a sample menu to get you started for a week:

Sunday	Monday	Tuesday	Wednesday	Thursday	Friday	Saturday
Rotisserie Chicken w/potatoes and broccoli	Boil chicken carcass for soup and add potatoes and corn for soup	Steak fajitas with peppers, onions and guacamole	Cut-up steak and add brown rice and Mexican toppings for a fiesta rice bowl	Breakfast for dinner with egg and cheese frittata and leftover vegetables	G.F. Panko crusted tilapia with broccoli slaw	Leftover fish taco on corn tortillas and guacamole

Common Food Items to Substitute

The following section is set up to give you a head start on what products I have found to be good substitutions in my recipes and lifestyle. I have tried these products and found them to work in my home, and this list will be a good place for you to start in building your own gluten-free pantry supplies.

Some of the brands in this section might not be available in your geographic area. It took me a long time and lots of money to try all these products, so it is a good jumping in point for you as well. You may find that you don't like, or can't find, some of the suggestions I've made, but certainly keep notes in this book to remember what you've experimented with. I've found that if you don't write it down, you will never remember.

Before you go and start throwing away the gluten-full foods in your pantry, here is a list of common foods that may contain gluten. Rather than throw them out, perhaps you can donate unopened items to a food pantry or give them to a friend or family member who can tolerate them. It's always good to familiarize yourself with this list so you can look out for them when you're not at home.

- Baking flours
- Breakfast cereals

- Pasta
- Bread
- Flavored rice and side dishes
- Crackers and snacks
- Breakfast items (pancake and waffle mixes)
- Pizza
- Cookies
- Breading and coatings
- Cake mixes
- Certain condiments
- Flavored coffee and teas (may contain barley malt as a sweetener, caramel coloring, or natural flavorings)

Where to Buy Gluten-Free Grocery Items

This is where my region might be different from yours, so be sure to make notes on the pages provided of gluten-free-friendly stores near you. Although different areas of the country have different specialty stores, many of the large national chain stores and online suppliers (Amazon) provide gluten-free grocery items. You can also find gluten-free products in places you would never think would supply them. Stores like TJ Maxx, Marshall's, Big Lots, and even the local CVS Pharmacy have shelves dedicated to gluten-free products, as well as organic and alternative grain products (i.e., almond flour, coconut flour, flour blends, etc.). I've found a lot of European brands or small batch providers that don't do large volumes of manufacturing that the grocery chains require at these types of stores.

Individual stores vary from location to location, so not all stores carry the same items. For example, the Giant brand grocery store closest to my home does not have a large selection of gluten-free products, but the Giant store ten miles north does. Talking with other gluten-free individuals and joining support groups is a wonderful way to find the small mom-and-pop stores that cater to certain brands you like. There are a large number of stores in Lancaster, Pennsylvania (Amish country), that carry unique, international, and gluten-free brands that I can't find at other stores. Shady Maple in East Earl in Lancaster County, Pennsylvania, is a perfect example. They have a huge international and organic section that has many gluten-free finds not available in my local grocery store. When I travel to Lancaster, I always stop at Shady Maple to see what new and unique GF products are in from all over the world. Many countries, like Israel, have products that don't contain gluten, so I love looking through the Ingredient list of products from that country.

Here is a list of Eastern regional stores that I find to have a good to great selection of gluten-free products:

- Wegmans
- Giant
- Redner's
- Kimberton Whole Foods
- Shady Maple

Large national chain stores that have a good selection are as follows (not in any order):

- Target
- Trader Joe's
- Whole Foods
- Costco
- Aldi
- Sam's Club
- BJ's

Notes about where to shop:

Gluten-Free Flours and Blends

Before I went gluten-free, I used to have one large bin of all-purpose flour in my pantry. It was fine for everything from cookies, cakes, and pies to pizza dough and breading. Of all the things to substitute in my pantry, I was confused most by which flour to use in place of my all-purpose flour. For as many alternate grains there are on the market (quinoa, brown rice, buckwheat, etc.), there are twice as many alternative grain flours and flour blends. I love to bake, so I was especially upset that I had to have so many different types of flours in my pantry (so I thought). Finding which ones work for different recipes is an art all in itself.

At the beginning of my journey, I started buying every type of gluten-free flour and flour blend I could find. I went to TJ Maxx and Home Goods and combed their shelves for unique and exotic baking flours. I would buy anything and everything and even try to make my own blends to bake with. Of course, I started out buying corn, potato, and rice flour. Then I found garbanzo bean, almond, and coconut flour. I became more courageous and bought sweet potato, sorghum, and tapioca flour. I tried blending flours and adding my own xanthan gum (gluten replacement) to make a replacement for good ol' wheat flour. Everything I tried failed because the flavors never resembled all-purpose wheat flour.

Then, from Northern California I found Cup4Cup flour blend. The famous chef Thomas Keller and his co-chef Lena Kwak developed Cup4Cup flour blend as a gluten-free alternative to use in any recipe that called for all-purpose flour. It was my first experience with using one type of flour for all my baking needs. Although many companies have come out with flour blends, I use Cup4Cup the most for my home baking.

Here is a list of other flours, along with Cup4Cup, and what I use them for. The products listed in **bold** (and throughout the Substitution section) are the ones that are currently in my food pantry now.

- **Almond (cookies and cakes)**
- Corn (coatings for frying)
- Brown rice (coatings for frying or thickening)
- **White rice (thickening)**
- Potato (thickening)
- Quinoa (baking)
- Sorghum (baking)
- Soy (baking)
- Sweet Potato (baking)
- **Tapioca (thickening)**
- Teff (thickening and baking)
- Amaranth (baking)
- Coconut (breading, baking)

Note: It's a good idea to keep flours in the refrigerator or freezer as they spoil quickly.

Brands of Gluten-free flour blends that I have tried for baking (they all work really well!):

- **Cup4Cup**
- **Bob's Red Mill 1-to-1**
- Arrowhead Mills
- King Arthur

Notes on flours and flour blends:

Breakfast Cereals

As healthy as I try to get my family to be, breakfast cereals is the one area we have the most arguments about. My daughter told our holistic practitioner that "the whole family has decided that Mom can't pick cereals very well and that Dad picks the good ones because they are not organic or gluten-free." Part of the problem, as my kids see it, is that my gluten-free cereals don't come with prizes, nor do they taste like they remember them. We have come to a compromise that they will eat "Mom" cereals during the week and "Dad" cereals only on the weekend. With that, I will tell you which gluten-free cereals I like and my children eat during the school week. There are also other national brands developing gluten-free cereal options.

Everyone has different tastes for cereals, so finding one that tastes familiar isn't hard, it's just finding what works for your family.

- **Gluten-free Chex brand cereals (Rice and Chocolate Chex are favorites)**
- Envirokidz Choco Chimps and Peanut Butter Panda Puffs cereal
- Van's Cinnamon Heaven
- Erewhon Crispy Brown Rice

- **One Degree Organic Foods Brown Rice Cacao Crisps**
- **Udi's, Chex, and LÄRABAR brand granolas**
- **Mom's Best Cereal (Crispy Cocoa Rice)**
- **Original, Honey Nut, Multi Grain, Apple Cinnamon and Frosted Cheerios**

Notes about cereals:

Pasta

My husband is part Italian (a "Heinz 57" variety of ethnicities). The Italian part is what makes him love his grandmother's secret spaghetti sauce recipe with rotini-style noodles. It takes days to make, and from my husband's perspective, tastes best when enjoyed over gluten-full pasta. He's been 100 percent supportive of my gluten-free changes in our house, but where baking flour was the hardest thing for me to substitute into our pantry, gluten-free pasta was my husband's—until Barilla came to the rescue. Their noodles hold up great smothered in red sauce or butter for the kids.

Before Barilla came out with their gluten-free version, I used to make two different pots of noodles for the family sauce, one with gluten-free noodles and one with gluten-full. Not only was it confusing to cook, but also my gluten-free pasta didn't really taste as good, especially the next day.

In my pantry, I had many different bags of noodles for different types of sauces. Corn pasta for red sauce, and rice and quinoa blends for pasta salads and white sauces. Our pantry was once again a testing ground for different types of noodles. Although I buy Barilla for standard Italian cooking, I have several Italian-produced noodles that I purchase when I find them on sale. Le Veneziane and Bionaturae organic pasta are two of my favorites. Both cook up perfectly and hold up into the second day better than others I've found. I can't always find them, but when I do, it's a treat.

I also found two brands of gluten-free pasta in the Jewish section of Wegmans grocery store during Passover. Although I haven't tried them yet, Manischewitz has a yolk-free noodle and Streit's has an Israeli couscous. Both are products of Israel and look like great noodle shapes to serve with soup. My husband just found a pasta on the Internet made in Italy by BiAglut, an H.J. Heinz Company. They have been making and selling gluten-free products since 1964, which was way before gluten-free was mainstream in the United States. Their products are available only in very specific stores, but they have a product finder on their website for convenience. I haven't tried it yet, but I'm excited to try something from Italy!

- **Barilla**
- Schar
- Glutino
- BiAglut
- Ancient Harvest Quinoa
- **Trader Joe's**
- Wegmans

- **Le Veneziane**
- **Bionaturae**
- **Simply Balanced (Target)**

Although I am forbidden from sharing the Arcara secret red sauce recipe, I do have an easy, delicious Alfredo sauce recipe to share in the recipe section of this book.

Notes on pasta:

_____

Breads

When I talk to people who mention they should be gluten-free they always say, "Oh, I can't give up my bread." My first reaction is, "If you want to get rid of that migraine, you would." But, then again, I forget how hard it was for me to find a type of bread that I enjoyed. Thinking back, I remember going to the local grocery store and buying some weird, spongy, tasteless bread from the small gluten-free/organic section. I paid a lot for that darn thing, so I was determined to choke it down, no matter how long it took. It took me months before I got through that first loaf and even longer before I found a different kind to buy. I didn't want to keep wasting my money on bad-tasting bread, so I took my time to find a new brand. It wasn't uncommon for me to stand in the gluten-free aisle and wait for people to walk up, just to ask them questions on what worked for them and what didn't. It was a great way to hear what people liked and were buying.

Bread is like cereal: everyone has a different preference to taste and texture. I like grainy bread for toast, so I found that Udi's is great for me and easy to find in most grocery stores (Target and Costco too!). If I am making a sandwich with untoasted bread, I look for Schar or Rudi's. For the family spaghetti dinner, I keep a baguette of Against the Grain and make garlic bread out of it. The Grainless Baker bakes a nice almond bread that I use on occasion, but my favorite breads are the ones you find baked locally and available at local farmers' markets or stores. What a treat to find something fresh baked.

Another great alternative to bread, believe it or not, is lettuce leaves. I have a celiac neighbor that swears she can roll anything into lettuce and eat it the same way as any bread sandwich. It's a great way to enjoy a burger or even chicken or tuna salad, and you get the nutritional benefits of eating some green leaves. I'm not saying that it's as enjoyable as a piece of bread, but it's certainly a good alternative if no gluten-free bread is available.

Below is a list of breads that are readily available and have worked for me. Breads are relatively expensive, so keep them in the freezer and look for them at the warehouse stores (Costco) to save some money by buying in bulk. Some gluten-free bread just tastes better toasted, so don't despair if you don't care for the texture out of the bag. Try toasting it to see if it works better for you. Also, Udi's and Schar make some good shape variations of breads (hot dog buns, bagels, sandwich rolls, etc.) that work for different recipes. By the way, a toasted Udi's bagel is great for pulled pork or a burger.

- Schar
- Glutino
- liveGfree from Aldi
- **Udi's**

- **Rudi's**
- **Against the Grain**
- The Grainless Baker
- Local bakeries (Amaranth Bakery, Betsy's Bakery, Sweet Christine's, etc.)

Bread notes:

Side Dishes

Many prepackaged side dishes are gluten-free and you wouldn't even realize it. Quinoa, rice, and even the stand by mashed potato are nice to enjoy. My favorite side dish is Lundberg brand rice products. They make a huge array of gluten-free rice products that are produced organically, sustainably, and they are committed to being non-GMO. Their mantra of "leave the land better than you found it" makes me want to buy the products even more. Many gluten-free products are listed on their website, and their products are easily found in any grocery store in the rice aisle. The only downfall of cooking rice is that it requires a little extra time to cook (up to fifty minutes). Some rice products are parboiled, so their cook time is greatly shortened. Lundberg also has quick-cooking flavored rice pasta dishes, lentils, and rice blends, which are always a good thing to have on hand.

Quinoa is another versatile grain that we eat often in our house. It easily picks up the flavor of whatever you cook with it. For example, add some cilantro and chili powder to make it Mexican or olives, garlic, and feta for a Mediterranean twist. You can even make it plain and eat it for breakfast with poached eggs. Its nutty taste and unique texture works well with fish, pork, chicken, or beef. I love its versatility, so I make a huge portion and use it through the whole week for any type of meal. Check out the great quinoa recipe in the recipe section to enjoy with dinner.

Instant gluten-free mashed potato flakes are always in my pantry. You never know when you might need a side dish and won't have time to make rice, or there is not a fresh potato in the house. They are convenient and quick, not to mention they are wonderful as a thickener for soups, sauces, and gravies. There are so many brands of instant spuds on the market, so I don't really have a preference. I don't use them very often, but they certainly are great in a pinch. I add fresh butter and a bit of heavy cream and it works for us! Just read the ingredient list to make sure it says "dehydrated potato."

A food that is a good side dish is macaroni and cheese. It can be a meal in and of itself, but I'm considering it a side dish for the sake of it. Hands down, my family likes Annie's Gluten-Free Rice Pasta and Cheddar. The flavor and texture is great, and for my kids (who grew up on Kraft), they really don't complain when I serve it. I find Annie's at our local Target store and always have a box on hand for a quick side dish or meal.

- **Lundberg brand gluten-free rice and side dishes**
- **Quinoa (Trader Joe's and Target's Market Pantry brands are good)**

- **Instant mashed potato (Wegmans, Idahoan, Betty Crocker, Hungry Jack)**
- **Annie's Gluten-Free Macaroni and Cheese**
- Trader Joe's Gluten-Free Macaroni and Cheese
- Seeds of Change brand rice and quinoa blends

Notes on side dishes:

Crackers and Snacks

This area of gluten-free food is changing constantly. New gluten-free crackers in different flavors (cheese, sea salt, onion, garlic, etc.) and other snacks are coming on the market every day. I love it! At the start of my journey, I could only find a few types of crackers, and they weren't always my favorite. But now there are so many flavors and textures to choose from that I can't even remember if I miss any of the gluten-full ones I used to eat. The manufacturers have gotten so good at using alternative grains for the products that my kids are eating more whole grains (quinoa, brown rice, oats) than before I went gluten-free. Our family prefers gluten-free pretzels to regular pretzels because they are so good. Glutino, hands down, has been our favorite pretzel. We've tried many different brands, but the flavor and texture of Glutino is the best. They are expensive, so I try to buy them in bulk when available at Costco, or even online from Amazon.

Nuts and seeds are another snack in my closet. I try to pound into my kids that they must eat a meat, cheese, or nut before they can have something sweet to get more proteins into their diet. With that, I keep all kinds of gluten-free nut bars (Kind, Luna, etc.) on the shelf as well as the whole nuts (pistachios, almonds, peanuts, and nut butters). How about popcorn? It's naturally gluten-free and is a whole grain. My suggestion is to look for organic and non-GMO corn and pop it yourself. Most microwave popcorn doesn't taste the same, and in my book, just isn't as good. Pop some seeds on your stovetop in coconut oil and sprinkle with Mediterranean pink sea salt for a special flavor!

Several household-name snacks that are not made with gluten or wheat ingredients find their way into our pantry. Cool Ranch Doritos are one of my son's favorite snacks, so on occasion I do buy them as a treat. My daughter is just like her mother and likes Fritos brand Cheetos. Believe it or not, they don't contain gluten or wheat ingredients either. As a matter of fact, many Fritos brand products are gluten-free. Their website has conveniently listed them for quick reference.

Remember Chex Mix? Yum! It is easy to make for a large group. It's also a perfect way to add some healthy options into your snack. Use gluten-free Chex cereals, and toast them with nuts (pecans, walnuts, almonds, etc.) and seeds (pumpkin, flax, sunflower, chia, etc.), and include some General Mills brand Bugles corn chips and gluten-free bagel chips to give them an interesting crunch. You don't need to rely on just prepackaged snacks to satiate your cravings. Be creative! Remember what I said earlier in the book? Use pre-packaged gluten-free foods as a vehicle to get something healthy and naturally gluten-free into your body.

Here's just a few of my family's favorite gluten-free snacks and crackers:

- **Pirate's Booty**
- **Tostito's Scoops (and corn chips)**
- **Food Should Taste Good brand chips and crackers**
- Lundberg brand rice cakes and chips
- **Glutino pretzels**
- Snyder's pretzels
- **Nuts, seeds, and dried berries**
- **Chex cereals**
- Bugles
- Gluten-free Cool Ranch flavored Doritos
- Fritos brand Cheetos
- Mary's Gone Crackers
- Van's brand crackers
- **Schar breadsticks**
- **Suzie's Thin Cakes (skinny rice cakes from Belgium)**
- **Mediterranean Snack lentil crackers**
- **Popcorn**
- **Breton gluten-free crackers**

The list goes on and on!

Cracker and snack notes:

Condiments

Condiments are a perfect example of all the odd places you can find gluten. When I started to learn about gluten, I visualized gluten as a binder for breads and baked goods. Then I learned that it was everywhere, including soy sauce. To say the least, I was in shock, mostly because I didn't even know I should be reading condiment and other liquids' labels to look for gluten-containing ingredients.

Another shocker was salad dressings. I just thought that salad dressings were made up of spices, oils, and vinegar. It wasn't until I learned *what gluten is* (refer back to step 1, "Elimination") that I realized gluten could be changed into a liquid form. The gluten protein from plants is not water-soluble; however, through a chemical process called deamination (Kalanick 2012), gluten is modified into a form that can be used as an emulsifier or thickener in liquids. By modifying gluten to contain less fat, it allows gluten to be used in another form and added into different types of products to give them new textures and structures. This is what allows salad dressings to stay combined and gives processed cheese its creamy texture. You can even see hair and skin products that contain gluten.

Deamination of the gluten protein makes condiments a hiding place for gluten (Kalanick 2012). I look for the words *caramel coloring* and *natural flavorings* in ingredient lists of packages. It is no wonder so many people suffer from unexplained digestive problems, not to mention other gluten-related symptoms (headaches, joint pain, sinus pressure, etc.). Gluten is all through food ingredient lists, so we are consuming so much more. You may think you are doing a good job avoiding gluten, but then you realize it's everywhere. Many students in my classes explain symptoms of fibromyalgia, depression, anxiety, migraines, brain fog, and joint pain while on (what they think is) a 100 percent gluten-free diet. At the end of my classes, students are often shocked at all the hidden sources of gluten that still need to be eliminated from their diet. Look for ingredient lists with the smallest amount of ingredients, or try to make your own salad dressing when you can. Condiments are a scary subject, so use the Internet if you are unsure.

I look for condiments that are labeled gluten-free to truly be safe or I go to the Internet if I'm not sure of any new products. Below are the items that I have in my pantry and refrigerator's condiment sections, but this is only a partial list of condiments you may need in your home. These are the items I have in the condiment section of my pantry and refrigerator.

- Tamari (gluten-free) soy sauce
- Worcestershire sauce (Lea and Perrins says it's GF on their website)
- Heinz ketchup and mustard
- Salad dressing (labeled GF)

- Tostitos brand salsa
- GF barbeque sauce (Sweet Baby Ray's)
- Pacific brand cream of mushroom and cream of chicken soup
- Pacific brand chicken, beef, and vegetable stock

Condiment notes:

Breakfast

Ah, breakfast foods…I could eat them for breakfast, lunch, or dinner. It's probably the easiest way to ingest clean foods with little preparation and little concern. Eggs, potatoes, vegetables—I can consume them all in an omelet and not worry about how it will affect me. With yogurt, fruit, nuts, or seeds, I can feel my body relax knowing that there is little chance of consuming gluten in those whole ingredients. My children are even comfortable making me breakfast since they can scoop out some yogurt and add some fruit with little or no worry. By far, it's my favorite gluten-free meal of the day.

I'm even finding that there are many tasty gluten-free breakfast items on the market. Gluten-free frozen waffles, cereals, bread, granola, and pancake mixes are just a few. Cooking them at home is the best way to prevent cross contamination, so I try to make meals at home as often as I can. However, there are several local places for breakfast that are careful to cook their pancakes in a separate part of the griddle than their coated hash browns, so this is another reason I feel comfortable eating out for breakfast more than any other meal of the day. Unfortunately, there is still one restaurant in town that will not accommodate gluten-free diners. They cook all over their griddle and when asked, the servers will flat out say, "There is nothing safe for you to eat here." That makes me sad because my kids love going there. But I do appreciate that the servers tell me, rather than me get sick.

Most other restaurants in town, if I ask, will be careful to cook eggs in a separate area of the griddle. Sometimes I order them poached. If I have time (and remember), I will bring my own gluten-free toast. The wait staff is usually not shocked, since many gluten-intolerant sufferers have been known to BYOSF (bring your own safe food) to enjoy.

Following is a list of what I have in my house now to enjoy for breakfast:

- Gluten-free oats (Bob's Red Mill and Chex brand quick oats)
- Gluten-free granola (homemade, Bakery on Main, Udi's)
- Gluten-free cereals (Chex, One degree, Envirokidz)
- Fruit smoothies
- Gluten-free baking mixes (Pamela's and GF Bisquick)
- Gluten-free frozen waffles (Trader Joe's, Van's, Wegmans, Eggo)
- Gluten-free toast (Udi's, Rudi's)
- Eggs (see my crustless quiche recipe at the end of the book)
- Jones Dairy Farm sausage
- Gluten-free labeled bacon (Applegate Farms)
- Grainless granola (LÄRABAR) with almond milk

Notes on breakfast:

Pizza

Friday pizza night at our local pizza shop used to be our family's best night of the week, until I went gluten-free. Then we stayed home, I bought frozen pizzas, and it was not the same. When Domino's Pizza announced that they had a gluten-free pizza crust, I loved it, but early on, I often got glutened by it. I found out that some stores would prepare and cook their delicious crust alongside all their gluten-full products. That is why I kept getting glutened. Pizza Hut (Udi's) and Domino's is now on board with a gluten-free pizza crust. I say, the more the merrier, just as long as they cook it safely (it's a learning curve for even these great companies).

Several make-your-own-pizza-crust mixes are on the market: Cup4Cup, Bob's Red Mill, Namaste, and Glutino. Even Taste of Home, whose products are sold through home parties, has come out with a pizza crust in a box. I must be honest, I haven't tried any of them, but I know they are available.

Finally, I found Sabatasso's frozen pizza at our local Costco. No kidding, we did a taste test at our house, and everyone liked the Sabatasso's pizza over many of the gluten-full frozen pizza brands. Another great idea is to use Udi's or Schar's premade pizza crust and add your own sauce and topping. It's fast and easy since the crusts are already parcooked. If we order a pizza to be delivered, I will use the Udi's or Schar and make mine to be ready when the gluten-full version arrives.

Friday night pizza is truly the one thing I miss the most about going gluten-free, but I would rather find a new pizza to enjoy than be sick. Following is a list of some pizza options for your Friday nights:

- **Sabatasso's**
- Against the Grain
- **Schar ready-made crust**
- Udi's ready-made crust or frozen pizza
- Amy's frozen pizza
- Freschetta
- Dominos
- Pizza Hut

Notes about pizza:

Cookies and Treats

Sometimes you just need something sweet and you want it now. I'm a certified health coach, and I have all kinds of suggestions for healthy, gluten-free, low-sugar treats. But sometimes, just sometimes, you want something quick, easy, and sweet and you don't have time to bake it. I also do not want a huge surplus of sweets in the house as a temptation.

Although I indulge in a prepackaged sweet on occasion, I don't make a habit of buying large quantities and keeping them on hand. For that reason, I like Schar brand products. They individually wrap small portion sizes, which allow me to have a sweet in my bag if the urge arises. There are many different flavors and brands of sandwich cookies. Trader Joe's and Mi-Del even carry a seasonal candy cane cookie (Oreo-type) during the holidays. I look forward to having that each Christmas as my special treat for the season.

Tate's and Trader Joe's also have crispy gluten-free chocolate chip cookies that taste as good as homemade. A friend of mine served Tate's ginger cookies at our church's Advent celebration, and everyone thought they were homemade. Another tasty cookie made locally in Eastern Pennsylvania is Bella Lucia pizzelles. They are quite pricy but come in several different flavors (traditional anise and vanilla) and are lovely to serve with ice cream for a special occasion.

I always keep a box of gluten-free graham crackers (for s'mores) or children's animal crackers on hand. Both are a delicious base for pies and bar cookies or as a quick snack for the kids. Most prepackaged cookies are expensive, so I use them sparingly and purchase those more as an addition to other desserts or as a special treat for myself.

When it comes to sweets, as I mentioned in previous chapters, prepackaged gluten free products tend to be higher in sugar and calories, and their portions are often smaller than gluten-full brands. Portion control is important when determining what to eat and how much you should eat. I'm one of those people who can eat one or two cookies and stop (my husband is not), which is what makes the Schar sandwich cookies nice since their packages are broken into small portions. It allows you to enjoy a small treat without having to open the entire package and letting some go to waste. In the recipe section of this book, I have a recipe for Mini-Energy Bar Treats, which are made with nuts, dried fruit, and chocolate. They are a nice treat to keep on hand.

Remember: *If you eat an entire box of cookies, gluten-free or not, you will gain weight.* So be mindful when choosing what and how many sweets to eat.

- **Graham crackers** (Kinnikinick, Trader Joe's, and Schar)
- **Snickerdoodles** (Trader Joe's)
- Sandwich cookies (Trader Joe's Jo-Jo's, Schar brand, Mi-Del)

- Pizzelle (Bella Lucia)
- Chocolate chip cookies (Tate's Bake Shop, Trader Joe's, Mi-Del)
- Snack cookies (Kinnikinick Animal Crackers)
- High-quality dark chocolate

Notes on cookies and treats:

Breading and Coatings

My kids love fried tilapia. Being able to say that about your ten- and twelve-year-olds is crazy, but we call it crunchy fish, and it's one of our family favorites (see the recipe at the end of the book). I buy the individually frozen tilapia fillets from Costco, so we can enjoy a few pieces at a time. I used to use gluten-full panko breadcrumbs, which puffed up in the oil and made a light crispy coating. It was one of those meals that my kids would say, "Please don't make this gluten-free. It just doesn't taste as good." How sad is that? So, I still make this dish, although it is difficult to prepare safely, both gluten-free and gluten-full.

As with any meal that you prepare gluten-free and gluten-full, you need to do the gluten-free preparation first, cook it in the oil first, and keep it warm in a two-hundred-degree oven. After you prepare your meal, clean the area and begin making the gluten-full version. It's a lot of work, but I do it because the kids really don't enjoy the gluten-free coatings as much on their fish.

When I started cooking gluten-free, most of the breadings were crumbly and were made mostly of corn. Honestly, they didn't produce the light crispy coating that made the fish so enjoyable. I tried to modify the gluten-free coatings using different kinds of breading and even added crushed tortilla chips and/or gluten-free crackers to try to come up with a new taste. It just wasn't the same, so I continued to make two versions of the recipe.

Finally, I found a brand of gluten-free panko-style breadcrumbs called Aleia's. It's got that great panko texture that I was looking for; however (as with most gluten-free products), it's more expensive. I've found over the last few years that there are so many good breadings available made with different kinds of grains. Corn-based breadings make great crispy coatings for chicken. Rice-based coatings, naturally, make a lighter, crispier coating for fish or as a topping for macaroni and cheese. I usually keep a corn and a rice breadcrumb mix on my shelf for different recipes. Believe it or not, gluten-free Bisquick is always convenient for quick recipes and serves as a base for coatings (and breakfast).

- GF cornstarch
- Rice flour or brown rice flour
- **Aleia's brand breadcrumbs**
- Kinnikinick breadcrumbs
- **Ian's Italian-Style Panko Breadcrumbs**
- **GF Bisquick**

Notes on breading:

_____

Cake Mixes, Baking Mixes, and Such

I cannot tell a lie…I love boxed cake mixes. Phew, that felt good to admit. Many gluten-free bakers roll their eyes when I tell them I don't make my own cake mix blends, but go for the convenience that a box cake mix offers. I guess it is because my mom always had a Betty Crocker or Duncan Hines boxed cake waiting for me after school. It was not only fast, but for a family of ten, it was economical as well. She wouldn't just make a cake—she would add bananas, chocolate chips, or take time to decorate the cakes to make them look fun.

Like my mother, I'm very creative with my boxed cake mixes. My secret is *The Cake Doctor Bakes Gluten-Free* by Anne Byrn. It has so many creative ways to bake and serve gluten-free cake mixes. Many of the recipes call for instant pudding, which gives the cakes a moist texture. A favorite in our house is Kathy's Cinnamon Breakfast Cake, which is a Bundt cake. It's moist, favorable, and really doesn't taste gluten-free at all.

There are so many good cake mixes and baking mixes on the market that it's hard to choose my favorite. I always have Betty Crocker GF Yellow Cake Mix on hand, but Wegmans GF White Cake Mix is perfect for special occasion cakes. I make the Wegmans cake, ice it with vanilla icing, and top it with toasted coconut. It's delicious and looks lovely as well.

Many different baking mixes on the market are also perfect for baking cookies, muffins, bars, and such. It's important to be creative in gluten-free baking without adding more sugar to the already sugar-laden ingredients. Using fresh ingredients in muffins, like strawberries, blueberries, nuts, or seeds, helps to add flavor and texture without adding more sugar. New Hope Mills makes a wonderful gluten-free blueberry muffin mix. When I'm going to a friend's and I want to bring these muffins as a treat, I make them with almond milk (to make them dairy-free) and coconut oil, and I top them with gluten-free oats, coconut oil, cinnamon, shredded coconut, and maple syrup or coconut sugar. Gluten-free or not, those muffins are wonderfully delicious!

Gluten-free prepackaged cake mixes are for convenience, so be creative and no one will know it's gluten-free!

- **Wegmans White Cake Mix**
- Wegmans Corn Muffin Mix
- Bob's Red Mill Brownie Mix
- **Betty Crocker Yellow Cake Mix and Brownie Mix**
- Arrowhead Mills All-Purpose Baking Mix
- **New Hope Farms Blueberry Muffin Mix**
- Aldi liveGfree brand brownie and chocolate chip cookie mix

Cake mix notes

Recipes

This book was not intended to be a cookbook (hopefully that will be coming soon!), but I wanted to include a sampling of some fun recipes that coincide with sections of the book. For example, the Alfredo sauce is great with gluten-free pasta, and the tomato recipe is a way to enjoy fresh, local ingredients. I tried to include a sampling of recipes that you can enjoy for breakfast, lunch, dinner, and a few snacks as well.

Alfredo Sauce

- 2 c. heavy cream
- 6 Tbsp. butter, cut into pieces
- 1 c. shredded parmesan cheese
- 1/2 tsp. grated nutmeg
- Dash of salt, pepper, and garlic powder
- Cooked chicken or leftover rotisserie chicken, if desired

Instructions

1. In a large saucepan on low heat, combine butter pieces and heavy cream by stirring constantly to prevent scorching.

2. When the butter is melted and combined with cream, stir in parmesan cheese.
3. Add nutmeg and salt, pepper, and garlic powder to taste.
4. Pour over gluten-free noodles and serve warm.
5. Add cooked chicken pieces or leftover rotisserie chicken, if desired.

Gluten-Free Cobbler

Berry Filling

- 3/4 c. coconut sugar
- 1/4 c. regular sugar
- 1–2 tsp. lemon zest
- 3 Tbsp. GF flour blend (Cup4Cup or Bob's Red Mill 1-to-1)
- 6 c. assorted berries, sorted, rinsed, and dried

Crumble Topping

- 1 c. GF flour blend (Cup4Cup or Bob's Red Mill 1-to-1)
- 6 Tbsp. sugar or coconut sugar
- 1 1/2 tsp. GF baking powder
- 1/4 tsp. salt
- 6 Tbsp. butter, chilled and cut into bits
- 1 large egg, beaten

- 1 tsp. GF vanilla extract
- 1/2 tsp. ground cinnamon combined with 3 tsp. of sugar
- 1/4 tsp. ground nutmeg, optional

Instructions

1. Preheat oven to 375 degrees. Butter a ten-inch round quiche pan or pie plate.
2. Berry filling: In a large bowl, combine sugar and lemon. Add the GF flour and whisk until combined. Evenly sprinkle mixture over berries in a prepared baking dish and toss gently. Set aside.
3. Crumble topping: In a medium bowl, whisk together GF flour, sugar, baking powder, and salt. Using a pastry blender, cut butter into flour mixture until it resembles a coarse meal with small, pea-sized pieces of butter.
4. In a small bowl, whisk vanilla into beaten egg. Using a fork, fold into flour mixture until moistened and dough starts to hold together. Don't overwork the dough.
5. Sprinkle crumble topping over fruit, and dust with cinnamon sugar and nutmeg.
6. Bake in preheated oven until golden brown and filling is bubbly, about forty to forty-five minutes. To prevent overbrowning of topping, cover with aluminum foil after twenty-five minutes.

7. Remove foil and transfer to wire rack to cool. Serve warm.

Crunchy Fish

- 3 Shallow dishes or pie plates
- 1 c. coconut oil or other high-heat oil, heated on a stovetop
- 3–4 boneless Tilapia fillets
- 1/2 c. GF cornstarch or rice flour for dusting
- 1–2 eggs, beaten
- 1 tsp. GF mustard
- 1/2 c. GF panko-style breadcrumbs

Instructions

1. Heat oil on stovetop.
2. Rinse and dry fish fillets.
3. Prepare three shallow dishes or pie plates to use for coating fish.
    a. Place cornstarch or rice flour in first shallow dish
    b. Combine beaten eggs and mustard in second shallow dish
    c. Place GF panko into third shallow dish
4. Dust fish in the first dish, cover with egg mixture in the second dish, and coat fillets with panko in the third.

5. Add the fish to the heated oil and turn over when brown.
6. Cook to an internal temperature of 140 degrees.
7. Serve warm with fresh cabbage and squeezed lime on a plate, or in a tortilla for a fish taco.

Crustless Quiche

- 1–2 Tbsp. olive oil or softened butter
- 2 medium shallots, finely chopped
- 8 slices of cooked bacon, crumbled, ham, sausage, or other cooked cured meat
- 1/4 c. grated parmesan cheese
- 1 c. grated smoked Gouda, Gruyère or Swiss cheese
- 2 c. half-and-half
- 6 large eggs, beaten
- 1/4 tsp. nutmeg
- Salt and pepper to taste
- Optional roasted red pepper, sautéed mushrooms, fresh spinach, or other vegetables

Instructions

1. Preheat oven to 375 degrees.
2. Sauté shallots in olive oil until tender. Add half of the cooked crumbled bacon. Remove from heat and set aside to cool slightly.

3. Brush a nine-inch pie pan with butter or butter-flavored cooking spray. Sprinkle evenly with grated parmesan. Add shallots and half of the bacon. Scatter half of the Gruyère and the remainder of the bacon.
4. Whisk half-and-half and eggs in a small bowl. Season with salt, pepper, and nutmeg.
5. Pour over filling and top with optional roasted red pepper and/or other vegetables.
6. Top with remaining Gruyère cheese.
7. Bake until the quiche is just set in the center, thirty to thirty-five minutes.
8. Serve warm with fresh greens or a side of fruit.

These can be made in cupcake pans and individually frozen to be enjoyed for breakfast on the go. Just heat them up in the microwave.

Homemade Hummus

- 1 c. dried chickpeas
- 2 tsp. baking soda
- 6 1/2 c. water
- 1 c. tahini
- 2 cloves garlic, crushed
- 4–5 Tbsp. freshly squeezed lemon juice
- Pinch of salt
- 6–8 Tbsp. ice-cold water

Instructions

1. First, soak your chickpeas in cold water and one tea-spoon of the baking soda the evening before (make sure to use twice the amount of water as your chickpeas as half the water will be absorbed). Soak overnight. Once your chickpeas are ready, add them to a pot, and add the rest of your baking soda. Sauté them for about three minutes. The baking soda will help break down the chickpeas and make them softer in your hummus.
2. Cover the chickpeas with water and cook them until they are soft enough that they can be easily squished in your hand. While they are cooking, remove any foam or skin that floats to the top.
3. Once your chickpeas are cooked, drain the water. Add them to your food processor. Run the food processor until they form a thick paste. Then add your tahini, garlic, lemon juice, and salt. Start pulsing with your food processor. Slowly add the ice water. Keep processing the hummus until you get a nice smooth, light paste.
4. Enjoy.

Mini Energy Bar Treats

- 2–3 Tbsp. local honey or good maple syrup
- 1–2 drops of GF vanilla extract

- 1/2 c. roughly chopped nuts (walnuts, cashews, pecans, almonds)
- 1/3 c. roughly chopped dried fruit (dried cherries, cranberries, or blueberries)
- 8-10 oz. high-quality dark chocolate, melted, to drizzle over top
- Pinch good salt (Himalayan pink sea salt)

Instructions

1. Combine honey and vanilla in a small bowl.
2. Layer minimuffin pans with chopped nuts and fruit, with honey mixture on top.
3. Drizzle a small amount of dark chocolate over the layers.
4. Sprinkle with a few pieces of salt.
5. Place in the freezer for ten minutes.
6. Transfer to a plastic container and place in the fridge.

Southwestern Quinoa and Kale Salad

- 1 c. quinoa, rinsed
- 8–10 oz. kale, cleaned and chopped into small pieces
- 2 Tbsp. extra-virgin olive oil or grapeseed oil
- 2 c. fresh or frozen corn

- 1 15 oz. can black beans
- 1 c. grape tomatoes, halved
- 2 Tbsp. fresh lemon juice
- 1 tsp. cumin
- 1/4 c. fresh parsley, chopped
- 1/4 c. pumpkin seeds or pine nuts, toasted
- Salt and pepper to taste

Instructions

1. Cook quinoa as directed. Allow to cool to room temperature.
2. In a large bowl, massage kale with oil to soften leaves. Add quinoa. Stir to combine.
3. Gently combine corn, black beans, tomatoes, and lemon juice in a separate bowl, trying not to smash the beans and tomatoes. Add cumin and parsley.
4. Fold the corn mixture into the quinoa/kale ingredients in the large bowl.
5. Sprinkle with toasted pumpkin seeds or pine nuts.
6. Add salt and pepper to taste.
7. Serve at room temperature.

Gluten-Free Stuffed Tomatoes

- 4 large or 6 medium tomatoes, insides removed and tops cut off

- 3/4 c. fresh or frozen corn, thawed
- 3 scallions, chopped
- 2-3 Tbsp. of olive oil
- 1 can 15 oz. black beans, rinsed and drained
- 1/2 c. sharp cheddar cheese
- 1/2 c. cooked brown rice or other leftover cooked gluten-free whole grain (quinoa)
- 1/4 c. gluten-free breadcrumbs
- 1/4 tsp. cumin
- 1/2 tsp. dried cilantro
- Pinch of Cayenne
- Salt and pepper to taste

Instructions

1. Cook corn and scallions on a cooktop over medium heat in 2 Tbsp. of olive oil until corn is lightly browned.
2. Wash and hallow tomatoes by removing the core and gentle scraping out the interior of the fruit. The opening should be large enough to stuff the tomato later. Try not to tear through the walls of the tomato.
3. Place hallowed tomatoes, right-side-up in a 9x11 oven safe casserole dish sprayed with non-stick cooking spray.
4. Add black beans, cheese, rice, half of the bread-crumbs, and spices to the corn until combined.
5. Gently add to hallowed tomatoes.

6. Sprinkle with remainder of breadcrumbs and drizzle with a small amount of olive oil.
7. Cover dish with aluminum foil and bake at 450 degrees for fifteen minutes. Remove foil and bake until browned on top.

Conclusion

Now that you have read my book, please don't stop there. Carry it with you. Write notes in it. Use it as a field journey for gluten-free shopping and eating. It's as easy as one, two, three, but in order to be successful, you need to keep notes of what does and doesn't work in your home.

Best wishes on *your* gluten-free journey.

Acknowledgements

I would like to thank my sisters and brothers (Michelle, Michael, Maria, Marguerite, Marcella, Suzanne [Sue], Mark, Matt, and Manette) for all their love and support. Every holiday is special because of the nine of you!

My sister Sue has always been there to watch over me, guide me, and be a positive role model and should have more than a paragraph written about how she diagnosed me with gluten intolerance.

To my wonderful children, Brendon and Katie, for being my gluten-free watchdogs and unofficial promoters of glutenfreebebe.com. You truly are the gifts that God has entrusted to me.

To my mother-in-law, Nancy, and all my nieces, nephews, in-laws, and out-laws. Thank you for always making something yummy to eat and listening to me talk about the benefits of being gluten-free.

To my amazing husband, Jeff. Without you, where would I be? You are my soul mate, and I am grateful for everything you have done to support me on my gluten-free journey. I could not have written *3 Steps to Gluten-Free Living* without you. Now I'm looking forward to helping you through your GF journey!

And finally, to my mum, Marcella. Your faith, love, and compassion have been my greatest examples through life. And to my dad in heaven, your voice rings in my ear, saying, "Grrrrrr! Savvy—do it now!" So I did, and this book is dedicated to you!

Melinda Arcara

aka Gluten-Free Bebe

(www.glutenfreebebe.com)

References

Alessio Fasano, M. 2013. "Why Creating the Healthiest Intestinal Environment Possible Can Arrest Your Vulnerability to the #3 Cause of Getting Sick and Dying." Interview by D.T. O'Bryan.

Amy Myers, M. "This Is Your Gut on Gluten." *Huffington Post*. http://www.huffingtonpost.com/amy-myers-md-/effects-of-gluten-on-the-body_b_3672275.html.

Anderson, J. *About.com*. http://celiacdisease.about.com/od/settingupthekitchen/tp/Make-Your-Kitchen-Gluten-Free-Six-Steps-To-Get-Rid-Of-The-Gluten.htm.

bakeinfo. http://www.bakeinfo.co.nz/.

Baker, B. *Eco Watch*. http://ecowatch.com/2014/04/29/fruits-veggies-dirty-dozen-clean-15/.

Celiac Support Association. http://www.csaceliacs.org/guide_to_oats.jsp

Celiac Support Association.com. "Grains and Flours Glossary" http://www.csaceliacs.org/grains_and_flours_glossary.jsp.

Celiac Support Association. http://www.csaceliacs.org/ csa_recognition_seal.jsp.

DrPerlmutter.com. http://www.drperlmutter.com/eat/ foods-that-contain-gluten/.

Freuman, T. D. *US News and World Report.* http://health. usnews.com/health-news/blogs/eat-run/2013/08/06/ making-sense-of-the-fdas-new-gluten-free-labeling-law.

Fugo, J. Gluten Free School. http://www.glutenfreeschool. com/2013/11/18/dentist-gluten-free-friendly/.

Gluten Free Drugs. http://www.glutenfreedrugs.com/.

Gluten Free Gigi.com. http://www.glutenfreegigi.com/ gluten-in-otc-and-prescription-medicines/.

Gluten Free Gluten.com. http://www.glutenfreegluten. com/articles/gluten-free-foods-list/.

Gluten Intolerance Group. https://www.gluten.net/ programs/.

Hill, M. American Chemical Society. http://www.acs.org/ content/acs/en/education/resources/highschool/

chemmatters/past-issues/archive-2011-2012/gluten.
html.

Hlywiak, K. H. 2008. "Hidden Sources of Gluten." *Practical
Gastroenterology*, 27-39.

Kalanick, D. B. August 6, 2012. *Better by Brooke. https://
betterbydrbrooke.wordpress.com/tag/inflammation/*
Retrieved April 8, 2015, https://betterbydrbrooke.word-
press.com/tag/inflammation/.

Klavinski, R. Michigan State University. http://msue.anr.msu.
edu/news/7_benefits_of_eating_local_foods.

Long, C. *Mother Earth News.* http://www.motherearth-
news.com/real-food/nutrient-levels-in-food-declining-
zb0z11zalt.aspx.

Long, C. *Mother Earth News.com.* http://www.mothere-
arthnews.com/real-food/nutrient-levels-in-food-declin-
ing-zb0z11zalt.aspx.

Luisa, C. *Natural News.com.* http://www.naturalnews.
com/035575_seasonal_food_diet_health.html.

McGinnis, J. *Natural News.* http://www.naturalnews.
com/032823_gluten_intolerance_celiac_disease.html.

National Foundation for Celiac Awareness (NFCA). http://www.celiaccentral.org/gluten-free-certification/.

National Foundation for Celiac Awareness (NFCA). http://www.celiaccentral.org/SiteData/docs/September2/35588e6068d17fe7/September%202013%20Webinar_Understanding%20...s%20Rule%20on%20Gluten-Free%20Labeling_Final.pdf.

Non-GMO Project.com. http://www.nongmoproject.org/find-non-gmo/search-participating-products/.

O'Brien, D. T. (2013). The Gluten Summit. Interview by M. Alession Fasano.

Patrick, S. *Gluten Intolerance School*. http://glutenintoleranceschool.com/gluten-intolerance-symptoms/.

QSRFoodNewsMedia.http://www.qsrmagazine.com/news/allergyeats-releases-2014-list-allergy-friendly-chains.

Rosenthal, J. 2007. *Integrative Nutrition*. The Donohue Group, Inc.

Schar.com. http://www.schar.com/en-us/gluten-free-living/gluten-freee-tips/cross-contamination-usa.

Teri Gruss, M. *About.com*. http://glutenfreecooking.about.com/od/gettingstarted/a/hiddengluten.htm.

The University of Chicago Celiac Disease Center. http://www.cureceliacdisease.org/.

Turbin, T. *Celiac.com*. http://www.celiac.com/articles/22706/1/Prices-of-Gluten-Free-versus-Regular-Foods---What-to-Do/Page1.html.

US Food and Drug Administration. FDA.gov. http://www.fda.gov/Food/ResourcesForYou/Consumers/ucm367654.htm.

50810071R00095

Made in the USA
San Bernardino, CA
29 August 2019